AF412909

CLINICAL PHYSIOLOGY SERIES

Physiology of Oxygen Radicals
Edited by Aubrey E. Taylor, Sadis Matalon, and Peter A. Ward

Effects of Anesthesia
Edited by Benjamin G. Covino, Harry A. Fozzard, Kai Rehder, and Gary Strichartz

Interaction of Platelets With the Vessel Wall
Edited by John A. Oates, Jacek Hawiger, and Russell Ross

High Altitude and Man
Edited by John B. West and Sukhamay Lahiri

Disturbances in Neurogenic Control of the Circulation
Edited by Francois M. Abboud, Harry A. Fozzard, Joseph P. Gilmore, and
Donald J. Reis

New Perspectives on Calcium Antagonists
Edited by George B. Weiss

Secretory Diarrhea
Edited by Michael Field, John S. Fordtran, and Stanley G. Schultz

Pulmonary Edema
Edited by Alfred P. Fishman and Eugene M. Renkin

Disturbances in Lipid and Lipoprotein Metabolism
Edited by John M. Dietschy, Antonio M. Gotto, Jr., and Joseph A. Ontko

Disturbances in Body Fluid Osmolality
Edited by Thomas E. Andreoli, Jared J. Grantham, and Floyd C. Rector, Jr.

Atrial Hormones and Other Natriuretic Factors

EDITED BY **Patrick J. Mulrow**

Department of Medicine
Medical College of Ohio
Toledo, Ohio

Robert Schrier

Department of Medicine
University of Colorado
Health Science Center
Denver, Colorado

AMERICAN PHYSIOLOGICAL SOCIETY
Bethesda, Maryland, 1987

PUBLICATIONS COMMITTEE

P. C. Johnson, *Chairman*
J. S. Cook
W. F. Ganong
L. R. Johnson
J. McE. Marshall

SUBCOMMITTEE ON CLINICAL SCIENCES

J. F. Biebuyck, *Chairman*
A. I. Arieff
H. A. Fozzard
P. J. Mulrow
N. B. Ruderman
R. W. Schrier
R. F. Zelis

S. R. Geiger, *Publications Manager and Executive Editor*
B. B. Rauner, *Production Manager*
L. S. Chambers, E. M. Cowley, S. P. Mann, *Editorial Staff*
C. J. Gillespie, *Indexer*

Preface

Regulation of blood volume involves complex homeostatic mechanisms, and control of sodium balance is a major contributor to this regulation. For many years the search for an elusive natriuretic factor was punctuated by exciting reports rapidly followed by discouraging negative results. The stouthearted continued the search and now have identified an Na^+-K^+-ATPase inhibitor that may originate in the hypothalamus. This inhibitor circulates in plasma, but its exact chemical nature is still a mystery. The last three chapters in this book describe the latest scientific findings in this tantalizing field.

More progress has been made with the atrial natriuretic factor. For over two decades it was known that distension of the atria of the heart caused a sodium and water diuresis. The mechanism of the diuresis was believed to be through a neural reflex and suppression of vasopressin release. It now appears that a peptide secreted from the atria into the blood contributes to the diuresis and natriuresis. This atrial natriuretic factor is known by several names: ANF, ANP, auriculin, atriopeptin, cardionatrin, and atrin.

The history of the discovery of this physiological system is most instructive. Granules were first noted in the atria under the electron microscope in 1956 by Kirsch. In the early 1960s it was recognized that these granules were similar to those found in endocrine secreting cells. Sporadic reports noted changes in the number of atrial granules in response to changes in sodium and water balance. The field lay relatively dormant until de Bold's classic experiment in 1981, in which he injected crude rat atrial extracts into rats and observed a diuresis and natriuresis.

In the short time since this discovery, remarkable progress has been made. The first section of this book describes the progress from characterizing the gene structure to measurement of blood levels in human disease. This new hormonal system has important actions besides its effect on the kidney: atrial natriuretic factor dilates blood vessels, inhibits aldosterone and renin secretion, and increases vascular permeability.

This book brings together for the first time these two important physiological systems: the Na^+-K^+-ATPase inhibitor and the atrial hormones.

Patrick J. Mulrow
Robert Schrier

Contents

Other Natriuretic Factors

1

Historical Perspectives of Atrial Specific Granules

ADOLFO J. DE BOLD

*University of Ottawa Heart Institute, Ottawa Civic Hospital,
Ottawa, Ontario, Canada*

THE DUAL CONTRACTILE-SECRETORY FUNCTION of muscle cells (cardiocytes) of the mammalian heart atria became apparent after electron-microscopic studies (1, 2, 14) that demonstrated that the bulk of these cells, unlike their ventricular counterparts, display a prominent Golgi complex, a large content of rough endoplasmic reticulum, and storage granules referred to as specific atrial granules (Fig. 1). This name does not reflect the fact that storage granules of the same nature are also present in the ventricles of nonmammalian vertebrates (3) and in other species such as elasmobranchs (4). Animals surveyed for the presence of specific granules include the shark, lamprey, hagfish, goldfish, frog, toad, turtle, chicken, flying squirrel, rat, mouse, guinea pig, cat, rabbit, dog, bat, hamster, pig, ox, and human.

The ultrastructural features of specific granules for the different species are generally similar in that they display an amorphous core, a limiting unit membrane, and may measure between 350 and 500 nm. The size and number of these granules vary amongst species and, in general, are inversely proportional to animal size. Thus atrial cardiocytes from large animals such as cows contain fewer and smaller granules than atrial cardiocytes from small rodents. This fact shaped much of the research on atrial granules: most of the investigations on these organelles have been carried out in small animals such as rats, which display many granules per cardiocyte. Nevertheless the atria of these animals are small, usually ~100 mg wet wt in an adult animal. The number of rats required in our laboratory from 1968 to 1983 to develop the different techniques referred to here, including the isolation work leading to the elucidation of the sequence of cardionatrin I, was close to 200,000.

Until the late 1960s, few techniques—other than electron-microscopic ones—were available to study atrial granules. Between 1969 and 1972 our laboratory achieved one of the first technical advances in the field, which consisted of the development of an isolation procedure for atrial granules, using preparative ultracentrifugation (5). This procedure was first used to demonstrate that rat atrial granules are not a major storage site for catecholamines, as some investigators previously suggested (16). After the discovery of atrial natriuretic factor (ANF) (6), the isolation procedure was used to assess the degree of association between this factor and the atrial granules (3).

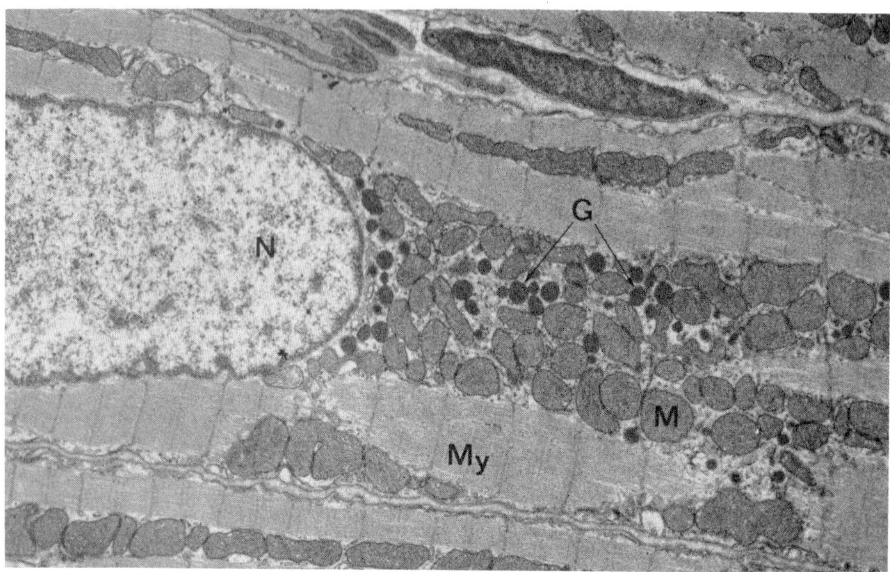

FIG. 1. Electron-microscopic view of paranuclear region from rat atrial cardiocyte displaying a modest content of atrial granules (G). N, nucleus; M, mitochondria; My, myofibrils.

It was found that 1) the highest specific natriuretic activity was associated with the purified granule fractions and 2) no fraction from ventricular muscle contained natriuretic activity.

Light-microscopic staining and histochemical investigations on atrial specific granules carried out during the mid-1970s in our laboratory (9) allowed for the development of an unbiased morphometric procedure to assess the degree of granularity of atrial tissue sections stained with lead hematoxylin (Fig. 2) and for the formulation of a hypothesis regarding the nature of ANF. Direct information concerning the development of an extraction procedure was also provided. Thus, before ANF was discovered, it was apparent that the atrial granules stored a basic polypeptide with a random coil conformation containing sulfur amino acids and tryptophan. Furthermore the diminished stainability of the granules after acetic acid–containing fixatives suggested formulation of extractants for ANF containing this acid.

One of the strongest indirect proofs of the relationship between atrial granules and ANF was obtained by determination of the natriuretic activity of extracts from hearts of different species (10). These investigations demonstrated that 1) there is a good correlation between the number of granules and natriuretic activity; i.e., the net specific natriuretic activity of extracts from atria known to have many granules (e.g., rat) is higher than that from extracts of atria known to have few granules (e.g., beef); and 2) in nonmammalian hearts the natriuretic activity is present, as are the specific granules, in both atria and ventricles. These investigations also hinted at a high degree of structural conservation for the atrial peptides because extracts obtained from different species were all found to be active in the rat bioassay.

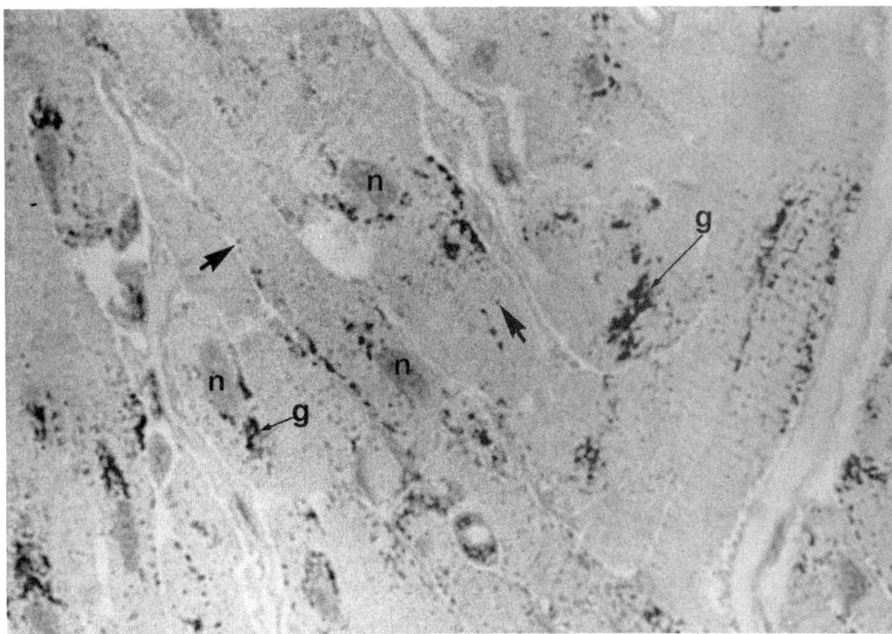

FIG. 2. Light-microscopic view of a 1-μm-thick section of plastic-embedded rat atrial myocardium stained with lead hematoxylin. Atrial granules are seen either singly (→) or in groups forming granulated areas (*g*). *n*, Nucleus.

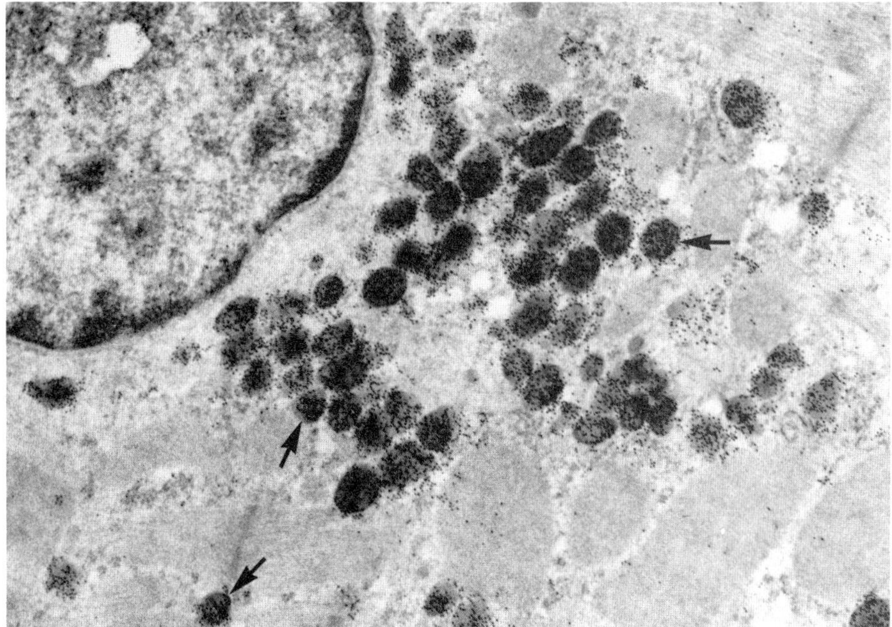

FIG. 3. Immunocytochemical localization of ANF in rat atrial specific granules (→) with the immunogold technique. Antisera used were obtained from rabbits immunized with synthetic cardionatrin I.

Further proof of a role for atrial granules as a storage site for ANF was obtained using the immunocytochemical approach (Fig. 3; 2, 8). Both light- and electron-microscopy immunochemical techniques using antisera raised against ANF peptides clearly localized these peptides within the atrial granules.

From the earliest studies on ANF (12) it has been apparent that this hormone is present in tissue as peptides of different molecular weights. Molecular cloning studies have demonstrated (see ref. 4 for a review) that, in the rat, preproANF is synthesized as a peptide 152 amino acids long. The most common tissue form, though, is a 126–amino acid peptide referred to as cardionatrin IV. However, the main released form is the 28–amino acid peptide cardionatrin I (7). Reverse-phase high-performance liquid chromatography of isolated granules or tissue extracts shows profiles that are very similar, in that the main immunoreactive form of ANF found in these extracts is cardionatrin IV.

From all of this evidence the function of the atrial granules is defined, approximately 30 years after their discovery, as the storage site for ANF in the form of cardionatrin IV.

REFERENCES

1. BENCOSME, S. A., AND J. M. BERGER. Specific granules in human and non-human vertebrate cardiocytes. In: *Recent Advances in Studies on Cardiac Structure and Metabolism*, edited by E. Bajusz and G. Rona. Baltimore, MD: University Park, 1972, vol. 1, p. 327–339.
2. CHAPEAU, C., J. GUTKOWSKA, P. W. SCHILLER, R. W. MILNE, G. THIBAULT, R. GARCIA, J. GENEST, AND M. CANTIN. Localization of immunoreactive synthetic atrial natriuretic factor (ANF) in the heart of various animal species. *J. Histochem. Cytochem.* 33: 541–550, 1985.
3. DE BOLD, A. J. Tissue fractionation studies on the relationship between an atrial natriuretic factor and specific atrial granules. *Can. J. Physiol. Pharmacol.* 60: 324–330, 1982.
4. DE BOLD, A. J. Atrial natriuretic factor: a hormone produced by the heart. *Science Wash. DC* 230: 767–770, 1985.
5. DE BOLD, A. J., AND S. A. BENCOSME. Studies on the relationship between the catecholamine distribution in the atrium and the specific granules present in atrial muscle cells. 1. Isolation of a purified specific granule subfraction. *Cardiovasc. Res.* 7: 351–363, 1973.
6. DE BOLD, A. J., H. B. BORENSTEIN, A. T. VERESS, AND H. SONNENBERG. A rapid and potent natriuretic response to intravenous injection of atrial myocardial extracts in rats. *Life Sci.* 28: 89–94, 1981.
7. DE BOLD, A. J., P. L. DAVIES, M. L. DE BOLD, T. G. FLYNN, B. P. KENNEDY, J. J. MARSDEN, I. R. SARDA, AND O. TADROSS. Morphological and biochemical aspects of atrial natriuretic factor (Cardionatrins). In: *Proc. NAITO Found. Int. Symp. Natural Products Biol. Activities, Tokyo, Japan*, 1986, p. 325–332.
8. DE BOLD, A. J., AND M. L. DE BOLD. Immunocytochemical demonstration of cardionatrins in human atrial myocardium. In: *Immunocytochemistry in Tumour Diagnosis*, edited by J. Russo. Boston, MA: Martinus Nijhoff, 1985, p. 202–206.
9. DE BOLD, A. J., J. J. RAYMOND, AND S. A. BENCOSME. Atrial specific granules of the rat heart: light microscopic staining and histochemical reactions. *J. Histochem. Cytochem.* 26: 1094–1102, 1978.
10. DE BOLD, A. J., AND T. A. SALERNO. Natriuretic activity of extracts obtained from hearts of different species and from various rat tissues. *Can. J. Physiol. Pharmacol.* 61: 127–130, 1983.
11. FLYNN, T. G., P. L. DAVIES, B. P. KENNEDY, M. L. DE BOLD, AND A. J. DE BOLD. Alignment of rat cardionatrin sequences with the preprocardionatrin sequence from complementary DNA. *Science Wash. DC* 228: 323–325, 1985.

12. FLYNN, T. G., M. L. DE BOLD, AND A. J. DE BOLD. The amino acid sequence of an atrial peptide with potent diuretic and natriuretic properties. *Biochem. Biophys. Res. Commun.* 117: 859–865, 1983.
13. JAMIESON, J. D., AND G. E. PALADE. Specific granules in atrial muscle cells. *J. Cell Biol.* 23: 151–172, 1964.
14. KISCH, B. Electron microscopy of the atrium of the heart. I. Guinea pig. *Exp. Med. Surg.* 14: 99–112, 1956.
15. SOLOMON, R., M. TAYLOR, D. DORSEY, P. SILVA, AND F. H. EPSTEIN. Atriopeptin stimulation of rectal gland function in *Squalus acanthias. Am. J. Physiol.* 249 (*Regulatory Integrative Comp. Physiol.* 18): R348–R354, 1985.
16. SOSA-LUCERO, J. C., F. A. DE LA IGLESIA, G. LUMB, J. M. BERGER, AND S. A. BENCOSME. Subcellular distribution of catecholamines and specific granules in rat heart. *Lab. Invest.* 21: 19–26, 1969.

2

Structure and Expression
of the Atrial Natriuretic Factor Gene

KENNETH D. BLOCH, J. G. SEIDMAN,
AND CHRISTINE E. SEIDMAN

Department of Genetics, Harvard Medical School, Boston, Massachusetts

HYPERTENSION AFFLICTS millions of people in the United States. In 90% or more of these cases, the etiology of the disease is unknown (38) and is referred to as essential hypertension. There is strong evidence suggesting that a predisposition for essential hypertension may be inherited, but the mode of inheritance is unknown (1).

Atrial natriuretic factor (ANF) is a circulating peptide hormone with a wide range of potent biological effects, including vasodilatation, natriuresis, diuresis, and inhibition of renin and aldosterone secretion (23). Atrial cells, which secrete ANF, are ideally located to detect and respond to changes in intravascular volume and blood pressure. Laragh (17) has suggested that a deficiency of ANF or a decrease in the response to ANF may be involved in some cases of essential hypertension, particularly those characterized by volume expansion.

The nucleotide sequence of the ANF gene has been determined, and the gene has been mapped to the short arm of human chromosome 1. Initial investigations of ANF gene regulation suggested that expression is relatively tissue specific and that ANF messenger RNA (mRNA) levels change in response to physiological stimuli.

This chapter discusses the molecular biology of ANF gene expression and the molecular probes available to assess the role of ANF in human disease.

STRUCTURE OF ANF MESSENGER RNA

The presence of secretory granules in atrial cardiocytes was reported in 1956 (16). Thereafter, several investigators observed that the number of secretory granules varied in response to changes in intravascular volume (5, 27). In 1981, de Bold et al. (6) prepared atrial and ventricular extracts and found that after intravenous injection into rats, only atrial extracts had natriuretic and vasoactive activity. By early 1984 several natriuretic peptides were isolated from rat and human atrial tissues (23). Sequence analysis of these peptides suggested that they shared a core of amino acids and were derived from a common precursor polypeptide. Collectively these peptides are termed *atrial natriuretic factors* (ANF).

To determine the structure of the ANF precursor, DNA sequences complementary (cDNA) to ANF mRNA were isolated. The cDNA "libraries" were constructed from polyadenylated RNA extracted from atrial tissues (19). The libraries were screened with synthetic oligonucleotides, representing all potential nucleotide sequences that could encode amino acid segments of ANF peptides. To increase the specificity of selection, oligonucleotides encoding two nonoverlapping amino acid segments were used. The cDNA clones, which hybridized to the synthetic oligonucleotides, were analyzed by nucleotide sequencing.

Nucleotide sequence analysis showed that rat ANF mRNA encodes a 152–amino acid precursor, preproANF (7, 13, 18, 35, 39, 41). Near its COOH-terminal, preproANF contains the amino acid sequences of ANF peptides isolated from rat atrial tissues (Fig. 1). The 24–amino acid hydrophobic leader sequence of preproANF may be involved in translocation of nascent ANF

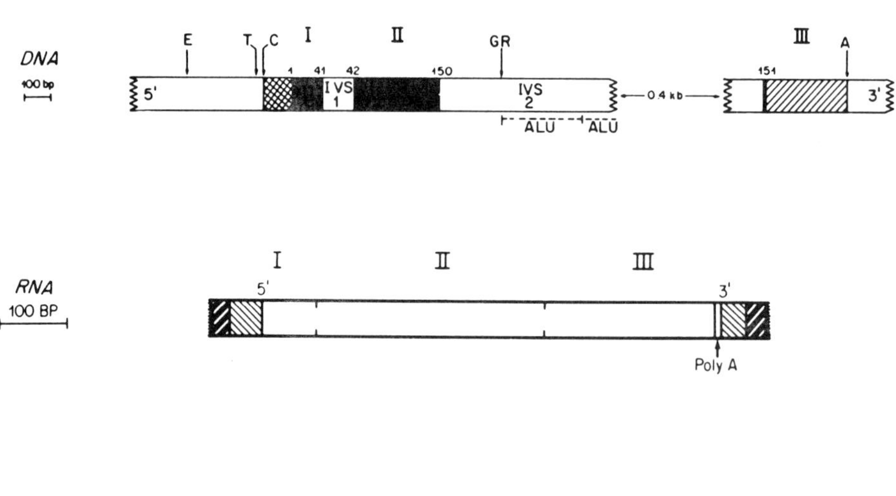

FIG. 1. Schematic representation of human atrial natriuretic factor (ANF) gene (DNA), mRNA (RNA), and peptide hormone (preproANF). Peptide coding blocks (I, II, and III) are separated by 2 intervening sequences (IVS 1 and IVS 2; IVS 2 contains reiterated *Alu* sequences). Putative enhancer (E), TATAA box (T), and cap site (C) are present at the 5' end of the gene. Potential glucocorticoid receptor–binding site (GR) and polyadenylation site (A) are shown. Processing of precursor ANF mRNA yields mature mRNA containing 5' untranslated sequences, joined coding blocks (I, II, and III), and 3' untranslated sequences. Translation of this mRNA produces preproANF. Hydrophobic leader segment and ANF peptide are indicated. bp, Base pairs; kb, kilobases. [From Seidman et al. (34). Reproduced by permission of the American Heart Association, Inc.]

precursor from the ribosome to the rough endoplasmic reticulum (33). By removal of the leader segment and the COOH-terminal arginine dipeptide, preproANF is converted to a 126–amino acid peptide, proANF. The predominant storage form of ANF is proANF (13); the circulating forms of ANF are derived from the COOH-terminal 28 amino acids of proANF (32). Atrial natriuretic factor mRNA has a 5' untranslated region ~90 nucleotides long, a 3' untranslated region 266 nucleotides long, and two AAUAAA polyadenylation signals.

The nucleotide sequence of a human ANF cDNA has also been determined (22, 27, 41). More recently, dog and rabbit ANF cDNAs have been cloned using the human ANF cDNA as a probe and their nucleotide sequences have been determined (26). Human and dog preproANF lack the COOH-terminal arginine dipeptide found in rat and rabbit preproANF: a single base change has converted an arginine codon to a translation-terminating codon. Rat preproANF contains a tripeptide sequence, Asn-Pro-Ser, that is not in human, dog, or rabbit preproANF and may be a glycosylation site. However, glycosylated residues have not been found in proANF isolated from rat atria (13).

REGULATION OF ANF GENE EXPRESSION

In atrial tissues, ANF mRNA is abundant, representing 1–3% of the total atrial poly(A)$^+$ RNA. As a first step toward understanding regulation of ANF gene transcription, the tissue specificity of ANF gene expression was investigated. To assess which tissues contain ANF mRNA, cellular RNA was extracted, fractionated on an agarose gel, transferred to a nitrocellulose filter, and hybridized to nick-translated, ^{32}P-labeled probe derived from the rat ANF cDNA (Northern blot analysis). Two groups of investigators reported that ANF mRNA expression was restricted to the atria: ANF mRNA was not detected in rat brain, liver, kidney, ventricular apex, aortic arch, carotid artery, pituitary gland, adrenal gland, pancreas, testes, epididymis, or hypothalamus (22, 34). In contrast, Gardner et al. (8) detected ANF mRNA in the ventricles, lung, pituitary gland, and hypothalamus of the rat, but at levels lower than those found in atrial tissues (i.e., ≤1–5% of atrial ANF mRNA concentration).

Extracardiac expression of the ANF gene is supported by immunohistochemical and biochemical analyses, which have demonstrated the presence of ANF peptides in the brain (21, 31), lung (30), and kidney (29). Failure to detect ANF mRNA in these nonatrial tissues may reflect insensitivity of Northern blot analysis (particularly if only a minority of cells in a given tissue contain ANF mRNA) or variation in ANF mRNA levels in different animal strains. Alternatively, ANF may be absorbed from the circulation and concentrated by ANF-binding sites in nonatrial tissues that do not synthesize ANF. In situ hybridization, a technique that may localize cells containing ANF mRNA in histological sections, should help distinguish these two possibilities.

To further study regulation of ANF gene transcription, changes in the concentration of atrial ANF mRNA in response to physiological and pharmacologic stimuli were investigated (Table 1). Nakayama et al. (22) observed atrial ANF mRNA levels in water-deprived rats. After two days of dehydration, ANF mRNA was decreased ~50%. Further decreases in ANF mRNA after four days of dehydration were accompanied by a depletion of total atrial RNA.

Takayanagi et al. (36) found a 70% decrease in atrial ANF mRNA in animals deprived of water for five days (measured by a quantitative dot hybridization assay). Concurrently, plasma ANF concentration decreased by 50%, while atrial ANF content increased ~200%. The latter finding is consistent with the observation that the number of secretory granules increases in the atria of water-deprived animals (5, 27). Although stringent dehydration decreases atrial ANF mRNA levels, the accumulation of peptide in secretory granules suggests that posttranslational controls are important in modulating plasma ANF concentrations.

The influence of dietary sodium on ANF production has also been examined. Takayanagi et al. (36) measured ANF mRNA levels in the atria of rats on high- and low-salt diets for two weeks. The concentration of ANF mRNA decreased in animals on a low-salt diet, but the concentration in animals on a high-salt diet did not differ from controls.

Administration of mineralocorticoids to animals causes transient fluid and sodium retention. Despite continued administration of mineralocorticoid, animals return to sodium balance within a few days, a phenomenon termed *mineralocorticoid escape*. To investigate the role of ANF in mineralocorticoid escape, Ballerman et al. (3) administered deoxycortisone acetate (DOCA) to rats in sodium balance and measured plasma ANF levels and atrial ANF mRNA content. Plasma ANF concentration and relative atrial ANF mRNA content (ANF mRNA compared with a constitutively expressed atrial mRNA species) increased in rats retaining sodium in response to DOCA. After "escape" from the mineralocorticoid-induced sodium retention, plasma ANF levels returned to base line while relative atrial ANF mRNA content remained moderately elevated.

Fluctuations in mRNA levels may significantly alter hormone availability for secretion. Conversely, given the high level of ANF mRNA in atria, peptide production may be independent of even dramatic variations in mRNA content.

These studies on the regulation of ANF gene expression have measured changes in the concentration of mRNA in atrial tissues. This technique does

TABLE 1. *Changes in concentration of atrial natriuretic factor (ANF) mRNA in response to stimuli*

Treatment	Concentration of Atrial ANF mRNA	Ref.
Water deprivation	↓	22
	↓	36
Low-sodium diet	↓	36
High-sodium diet	no change	36
Deoxycortisone acetate	↑	3

not distinguish between changes in ANF gene transcription and changes in the stability of the ANF mRNA.

There is considerable evidence that the primary stimulus for ANF secretion from cardiocytes is atrial distension (24). Atrial "stretch" may alter ANF mRNA levels by depletion of atrial stores of ANF, which might serve as a stimulus for increased ANF gene expression or mRNA stability. Alternatively, a mechanical stimulus, atrial stretch, may be transduced via an intracellular second messenger to change the rate of atrial ANF mRNA transcription or degradation. The mineralocorticoid-induced increase in ANF mRNA might occur as a result of sodium retention and atrial stretch, or it might represent a direct augmentation of ANF mRNA stability or transcription [perhaps via a steroid hormone receptor binding to the ANF gene (10, 33)].

STRUCTURE OF THE ANF GENE

To understand the molecular regulation of ANF gene transcription as well as the tissue specificity of transcription, reseachers cloned the genes encoding the human (10, 25, 33), rat (2), and mouse (33) ANF genes and determined their nucleotide sequences. Southern blot analysis utilizing the ANF cDNA to probe genomic DNA digested with restriction enzymes suggests that there is a single ANF gene in rodents and humans (25, 26, 35).

The ANF gene was isolated from human, rat, and mouse genomic libraries, with a rat ANF cDNA as a probe. Nucleotide sequence analysis of these genes revealed that each has three coding regions (exons) and two intervening sequences (introns) (Fig. 1). The first exon encodes a hydrophobic leader segment and the first 16 amino acids of proANF. The second exon contains the remaining coding information for proANF except for one amino acid in humans and three residues in rodents. These COOH-terminal amino acids are encoded in the third exon. The second intervening sequence of the human gene contains two tandem reiterated sequences highly homologous to a consensus *Alu* sequence (10, 25, 33).

The ANF gene has many features common to all eucaryotic genes, including a TATAA box (A, adenine; T, thymine), a consensus sequence found in promoter regions; intervening sequences bounded by GT-AG splicing signals (G, guanine); and AATAAA polyadenylation addition signals. Transcription start sites for the human (22, 25) and rat (18, 39) mRNAs have been investigated by primer extension techniques and are located ~30 base pairs 3' to the respective TATAA boxes.

Because ANF is probably critical in the regulation of intravascular volume homeostasis (24), mutations in the ANF gene that adversely affect the production of biologically active ANF could place the organism at a disadvantage and might therefore be lost during evolution. Conversely, sequences important for regulation of ANF gene transcription and production of a functional hormone would be expected to be conserved in the human and rodent genomes as these species diverged during evolution. Genomic nucleotide sequences from several species were compared to identify conserved regions. Comparison of the nucleotide sequences of the mouse and rat genes revealed marked conservation throughout, a finding that is consistent with the expected genetic similarity of closely related species. Comparison of the nucleotide sequences of human and rodent, species that diverged evolutionarily 70 million years ago (4), revealed specific regions of conservation and diversity (Fig. 2).

Sequences 5' to the transcription start site are highly conserved in all three species; the homology extends to the limits of nucleotide sequence data. As these sequences may be responsible for regulating transcription of the ANF gene, they were screened for homology to previously identified regulatory sequences. "Enhancers" are *cis*-acting sequences present in certain viral and eucaryotic genomes that augment the level of transcription of promoter regions that occur near them. The function of some enhancers is tissue specific. Although a consensus sequence for enhancer elements has not been defined, enhancers from some genes share sequences with the viral simian virus 40 (SV40) enhancer (15). Sequences in the 5' flanking regions of ANF genes are identical to a portion of the SV40 enhancer at 9 of 11 (human and rat) and 8 of 11 (mouse) base pairs. Perhaps these enhancerlike sequences are responsible for the high level of ANF transcription in atria. The biological activity of these enhancerlike sequences has not been determined.

The sequences encoding preproANF are more highly conserved between human and rodent genes than are the intervening sequences or the 5' and 3' untranslated sequences. Comparison of the human, rat, and mouse genomic sequences and rabbit and dog cDNAs demonstrates maximum homology in the regions encoding proANF (93 of 126 amino acid residues are identical in all 5 species). Less homology is evident in the hydrophobic leader segments (6 of 25 residues are identical) (26). Specific amino acids may be less important than regional hydrophobicity for the function of the leader segment (33).

The circulating forms of ANF are derived from the COOH-terminal amino

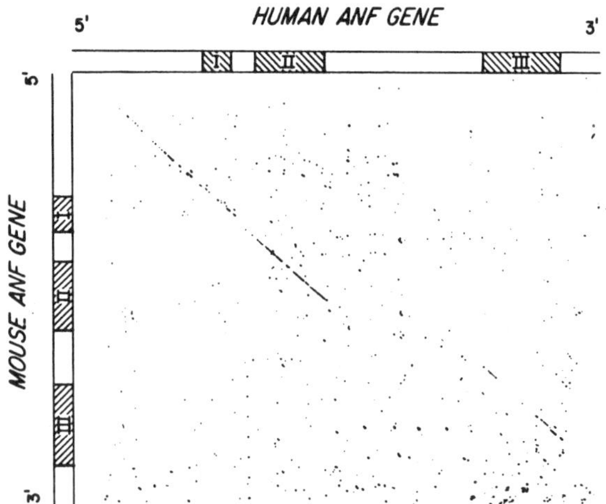

FIG. 2. Dot matrix comparison of human and mouse ANF genes. A single dot represents a base pair where 10 of 15 of the surrounding bases are identical between mouse and human genes. Line made of dots, region of extensive homology. [From Seidman et al. (34). Reproduced by permission of the American Heart Association, Inc.]

acids of proANF (32). Marked nucleotide and amino acid homology between species suggests that biological activity of the hormone would be adversely affected by diversity. The function of the amino acids at the NH_2-terminal of proANF is unknown; however, the extensive nucleotide and amino acid sequence homology among divergent species suggests a biologically important role. Demonstration of multiple biologically active peptides within a single hormone precursor, e.g., pro-opiomelanocortin (12), led investigators to speculate that processing of proANF generates physiologically important peptides from the NH_2-terminal of proANF (22). Alternatively, the NH_2-terminal of proANF may play a role in packaging of proANF into secretory granules.

A nucleotide sequence present in the second intervening sequence of the human ANF gene is identical to a consensus sequence for the glucocorticoid receptor–binding site (14) at 9 of 11 base pairs (10, 33). The mouse and rat ANF genes lack this sequence. Human growth hormone gene contains a functional glucocorticoid receptor–binding site that is absent in the mouse gene (20). The biological activity of the potential glucocorticoid receptor–binding site in the human ANF gene is undetermined.

GENETIC LINKAGE STUDIES

Molecular mechanisms regulating transcription of the ANF gene can be studied by identification of human or animal phenotypes that are the result of mutations in the ANF gene. For example, a mutation in the promoter region of the ANF gene could result in decreased atrial ANF mRNA, decreased ANF secretion, and volume expansion and might present clinically as hypertension. Mutations in the peptide-encoding sequences could result in defective circulating ANF or in abnormal processing of proANF. No disease states associated with a deficiency or abnormality in ANF have been clearly identified. As an alternative, examination of the genetic linkage of the ANF gene with disease states may permit identification of genetic disorders whose biochemical etiology is unknown.

A first approach to identifying diseases that are linked to the ANF gene is to investigate the surrounding genetic map. Yang-Feng et al. (40) have performed chromosomal localization of the ANF gene in human and mouse genomes. In situ hybridization to human chromosomes, with a ^{3}H-labeled human ANF probe, labeled the short arm of chromosome 1, band p36 (subband 1p36.2). This result was confirmed by Southern blot analysis of human × Chinese hamster somatic cell hybrids. Positive hybridization occurred only with those somatic cell hybrids containing the 1p32→1pter portion of human chromosome 1. Similarly, Southern blot analysis of mouse × Chinese hamster somatic cell hybrid DNA permitted localization of the ANF gene to mouse chromosome 4. Knowledge of the chromosomal map surrounding the ANF gene may be useful for the identification of diseases related to ANF.

Restriction fragment-length polymorphisms (RFLPs) can be used to link genes with disease states: RFLPs also reflect allelic differences in nucleotide sequences, which may be identified by restriction enzymes and appropriate DNA probes. Analysis of RFLPs has been used to study the linkage of familial hypoalphalipoproteinemia, a disorder characterized by premature atherosclerosis, with the apolipoprotein A-I gene (28). Nemer et al. (25) observed allelic variation in two human ANF cDNA clones: one of two base-pair differences resulted in the presence of a new *Kpn*I restriction enzyme cleavage site and the extension of the encoded ANF precursor by two arginine residues. (This base-pair difference might be identified by the loss of an *Sca*I restriction enzyme cleavage site in genomic DNA.) No disease state has been correlated with this polymorphism.

Graham et al. (9) investigated the potential linkage of the ANF gene with Bartter's syndrome, a rare fluid and electrolyte disorder characterized by hyperreninemia, hypokalemic alkalosis, and growth retardation. Although most cases of Bartter's syndrome are sporadic, familial cases have suggested an autosomal recessive mode of inheritance. Overproduction of an unknown natriuretic substance has been proposed as the etiology of Bartter's syndrome (11). Because ANF has potent natriuretic properties, it was considered a prime candidate for the unknown natriuretic substance.

Graham et al. (9) extracted DNA from the blood of members of a large kindred with six affected members (Fig. 3). An RFLP in the ANF gene was identified in one of two alleles of the male member in the first generation. If Bartter's syndrome is caused by an abnormality of the ANF gene, inheritance of one of the two ANF alleles should closely correlate with inheritance of the disease. Analysis of RFLPs of DNAs from the second generation demonstrated that neither allele cosegregated with clinical evidence of Bartter's syndrome. Hence, in this kindred, the ANF gene is not genetically linked to Bartter's syndrome.

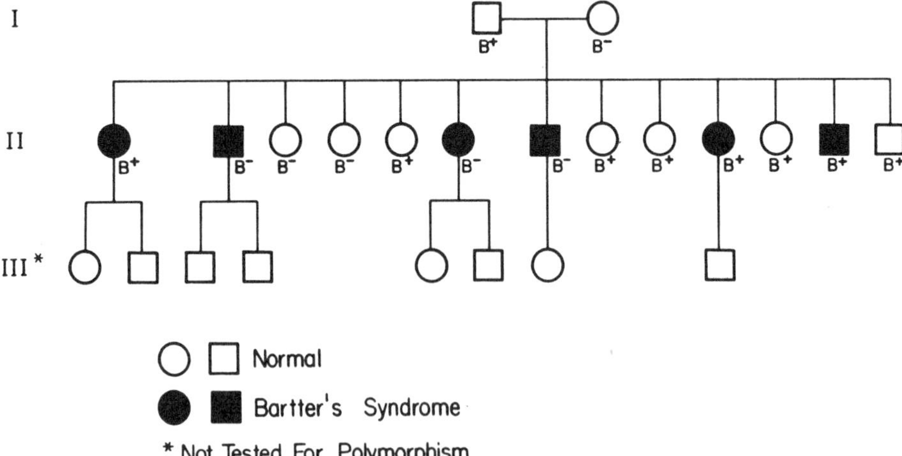

FIG. 3. Family pedigree. Segregation of Bartter's syndrome and presence (B$^+$) or absence (B$^-$) of an ANF gene polymorphism. [From Graham et al. (9). Reproduced by permission of the American Heart Association, Inc.]

Although the evaluation of the possible genetic linkage of the ANF gene and Bartter's syndrome produced a negative result, it illustrates the potential usefulness of RFLP analysis in understanding a genetic basis of fluid and electrolyte disorders.

CONCLUSIONS

Atrial natriuretic factor is a cardiac hormone with potent natriuretic, diuretic, and vasorelaxant activities. Amino acid sequence analysis of this peptide has permitted application of molecular techniques to construct a cDNA corresponding to ANF mRNA and to define and characterize the ANF gene. Genetic probes have provided insights into the regulation of hormone production and may help define genetic etiologies of human disease.

We acknowledge the contributions of our collaborators: Jerome B. Zisfein, John A. Smith, Edgar Haber, Charles J. Homcy, and Robert M. Graham.

Research from our laboratory was supported by a fellowship from the Leukemia Society of America, Inc. (KDB), a fellowship from the Mallinkrodt Foundation, and National Institutes of Health Grants AI-18436 (JGS) and HL-35642 (CES and JGS).

REFERENCES

1. ALFREY, A. Renal responses to vascular injury. In: *The Kidney*, edited by B. M. Brenner and F. C. Rector. Philadelphia, PA: Saunders, 1981, p. 1668–1718.
2. ARGENTIN, S., M. NEMER, J. DROUIN, G. K. SCOTT, B. P. KENNEDY, AND P. L. DAVIES. The gene for rat atrial natriuretic factor. *J. Biol. Chem.* 260: 4568–4571, 1985.
3. BALLERMAN, B. J., K. D. BLOCH, J. G. SEIDMAN, AND B. M. BRENNER. Atrial natriuretic peptide transcription, secretion, and glomerular receptor activity during mineralocorticoid escape. *J. Clin. Invest.* 78: 840–843, 1986.
4. DAYHOFF, M. O. *Atlas of Protein Sequence and Structure.* Silver Spring, MD: Natl. Biomed. Res. Found., 1965.
5. DE BOLD, A. J. Atrial natriuretic factor: a hormone produced by the heart. *Science Wash. DC* 230: 767–770, 1985.
6. DE BOLD, A. J., H. B. BORENSTEIN, A. T. VERESS, AND H. SONNENBERG. A rapid and potent natriuretic response to intravenous injection of atrial myocardial extracts in rats. *Life Sci.* 28: 89–94, 1981.
7. FLYNN, T. G., P. L. DAVIES, B. P. KENNEDY, M. L. DE BOLD, AND A. J. DE BOLD. Alignment of rat cardionatrin sequences with the preprocardionatrin sequence from complementary DNA. *Science Wash. DC* 228: 323–325, 1985.
8. GARDNER, D. G., J. A. LEWICKI, J. C. FIDDES, C. H. METZLER, D. J. RAMSAY, D. TRACHEWSKY, S. HANE, AND J. D. BAXTER. Preauriculin gene expression: detection in extraatrial tissues and regulation of cardiac and extracardiac mRNA levels by glucocorticoids and mineralocorticoids (abstr.). *Clin. Res.* 33: 553A, 1985.
9. GRAHAM, R. M., K. D. BLOCH, V. B. DELANEY, E. BOURKE, AND J. G. SEIDMAN. Bartter's syndrome and the atrial natriuretic factor gene. *Hypertension Dallas* 8: 549–551, 1986.
10. GREENBERG, B. D., G. H. BENCEN, J. J. SEILHAMER, J. A. LEWICKI, AND J. C. FIDDES. Nucleotide sequence of the gene encoding human atrial natriuretic factor precursor. *Nature Lond.* 312: 656–658, 1984.
11. GREKIN, R. J., M. G. NICHOLLS, AND P. L. PADFIELD. Disorders of chloriuretic hormone secretion. *Lancet* 1: 1116–1118, 1979.
12. HABENER, J. F., P. K. LUND, J. W. JACOBS, P. C. DEE, AND R. H. GOODMAN. Polyprotein precursors of regulatory peptides. In: *Peptides: Synthesis-Structure-Function*, edited by D. H. Rich and E. Gross. Rockford, IL: Pierce Chem., 1981, p. 457–469. (Proc. 7th Am. Pept. Symp.)

13. KANGAWA, K., Y. TAWARAGI, S. OIKAWA, A. MIZUNO, Y. SAKURAGAWA, H. NAKAZATO, A. FUKUDA, N. MINAMINO, AND H. MATSUO. Identification of rat γ atrial natriuretic polypeptide and characterization of the cDNA encoding its precursor. *Nature Lond.* 312: 152–155, 1984.

14. KARIN, M., A. HASLINGER, H. HOLTGREVE, R. I. RICHARDS, P. KRAUTER, H. M. WESTPHAL, AND M. BEATO. Characterization of DNA sequences through which cadmium and glucocorticoid hormones induce human metallothionein-II$_A$ gene. *Nature Lond.* 308: 513–519, 1984.

15. KHOURY, G., AND P. GRUSS. Enhancer elements. *Cell* 33: 313–314, 1983.

16. KIRSH, B. Electron microscopy of the atrium of the heart. I. Guinea pig. *Exp. Med. Surg.* 114: 99–112, 1956.

17. LARAGH, J. Atrial natriuretic hormone, the renin-aldosterone axis, and blood pressure-electrolyte homeostasis. *N. Engl. J. Med.* 313: 1330–1340, 1985.

18. MAKI, M., R. TAKAYANAGI, K. S. MISONO, K. N. PANDEY, C. TIBBETTS, AND T. INAGAMI. Structure of rat atrial natriuretic factor precursor deduced from cDNA sequence. *Nature Lond.* 309: 722–724, 1984.

19. MANIATIS, T., E. F. FRITSCH, AND J. SAMBROOK. *Molecular Cloning: A Laboratory Manual.* Cold Spring Harbor, NY: Cold Spring Harbor, 1982.

20. MOORE, D. D., A. R. MARKS, D. I. BUCKLEY, G. KAPLER, F. PAYVAR, AND H. M. GOODMAN. The first intron of the human growth hormone gene contains a binding site for glucocorticoid receptor. *Proc. Natl. Acad. Sci. USA* 82: 699–702, 1985.

21. MORII, N., K. NAKAO, A. SUGAWARA, M. SAKAMOTO, M. SUDA, M. SHIMOKURA, Y. KISO, M. KIHARA, Y. YAMORI, AND H. IMURA. Occurrence of atrial natriuretic polypeptide in brain. *Biochem. Biophys. Res. Commun.* 127: 413–419, 1985.

22. NAKAYAMA, K., H. OHKUBO, T. HIROSE, S. INAYAMA, AND S. NAKANISHI. mRNA sequence for human cardiodilatin-atrial natriuretic factor precursor and regulation of precursor mRNA in rat atria. *Nature Lond.* 310: 699–701, 1984.

23. NEEDLEMAN, P., S. P. ADAMS, B. R. COLE, M. G. CURRIE, D. M. GELLER, M. L. MICHENER, C. B. SAPER, D. SCHWARTZ, AND D. G. STANDAERT. Atriopeptins as cardiac hormones. *Hypertension Dallas* 7: 469–482, 1985.

24. NEEDLEMAN, P., AND J. E. GREENWALD. Atriopeptin: a cardiac hormone intimately involved in fluid, electrolyte, and blood-pressure homeostasis. *N. Engl. J. Med.* 314: 828–833, 1986.

25. NEMER, M., M. CHAMBERLAND, D. SIROIS, S. ARGENTIN, J. DROUIN, R. A. DIXON, R. A. ZIVIN, AND J. H. CONDRA. Gene structure of human cardiac hormone precursor, pronatriodilatin. *Nature Lond.* 312: 654–656, 1984.

26. OIKAWA, S., M. IMAI, C. INUZUKA, Y. TAWARAGI, H. NAKAZATO, AND H. MATSUO. Structure of dog and rabbit precursors of atrial natriuretic polypeptides deduced from nucleotide sequence of cloned cDNA. *Biochem. Biophys. Res. Commun.* 132: 892–899, 1985.

27. OIKAWA, S., M. IMAI, A. UENO, S. TANAKA, T. NOGUCHI, H. NAKAZATO, K. KANGAWA, A. FUKUDA, AND H. MATSUO. Cloning and sequence analysis of cDNA encoding a precursor for human atrial natriuretic polypeptide. *Nature Lond.* 309: 724–726, 1984.

28. ORDOVAS, J. M., E. J. SCHAEFER, D. SALEM, R. H. WARD, C. J. GLUECK, C. VERGANI, P. W. F. WILSON, AND S. K. KARATHANASIS. Apolipoprotein A-I gene polymorphism associated with premature coronary artery disease and familial hypoalphalipoproteinemia. *N. Engl. J. Med.* 314: 671–677, 1986.

29. SAKAMOTO, M., K. NAKAO, M. KIHARA, N. MORII, A. SUGAWARA, M. SUDA, M. SHIMOKURA, Y. KISO, Y. YAMORI, AND H. IMURA. Existence of atrial natriuretic polypeptide in kidney. *Biochem. Biophys. Res. Commun.* 128: 1281–1287, 1985.

30. SAKAMOTO, M., K. NAKAO, N. MORII, A. SUGAWARA, T. YAMADA, H. ITOH, S. SHIONO, Y. SAITO, AND H. IMURA. The lung as a possible target organ for atrial natriuretic polypeptide secreted from the heart. *Biochem. Biophys. Res. Commun.* 135: 515–520, 1985.

31. SAPER, C. B., D. G. STANDAERT, M. G. CURRIE, D. SCHWARTZ, D. M. GELLER, AND P. NEEDLEMAN. Atriopeptin-immunoreactive neurons in the brain: presence in cardiovascular regulatory areas. *Science Wash. DC* 227: 1047–1049, 1985.

32. SCHWARTZ, D., D. M. GELLER, P. T. MANNING, N. R. SIEGEL, K. F. FOK, C. E. SMITH, AND P. NEEDLEMAN. Ser-Leu-Arg-Arg-atriopeptin III: the major circulating form of atrial peptide. *Science Wash. DC* 229: 397–400, 1985.

33. SEIDMAN, C. E., K. D. BLOCH, K. A. KLEIN, J. A. SMITH, AND J. G. SEIDMAN. Nucleotide sequences of the human and mouse atrial natriuretic factor genes. *Science Wash. DC* 226: 1206–1209, 1984.

34. SEIDMAN, C. E., K. D. BLOCH, J. ZISFEIN, J. A. SMITH, E. HABER, C. HOMCY, A. D. DUBY,

E. CHOI, R. M. GRAHAM, AND J. G. SEIDMAN. Molecular studies of the atrial natriuretic factor gene. *Hypertension Dallas* 7, Suppl. I: 31–34, 1985.

35. SEIDMAN, C. E., A. D. DUBY, E. CHOI, R. M. GRAHAM, E. HABER, C. HOMCY, J. A. SMITH, AND J. G. SEIDMAN. The structure of rat preproatrial natriuretic factor as defined by a complementary DNA clone. *Science Wash. DC* 225: 324–326, 1984.

36. TAKAYANAGI, R., I. TANAKA, M. MAKI, AND T. INAGAMI. Effects of changes in water-sodium balance on levels of atrial natriuretic factor messenger RNA and peptide in rats. *Life Sci.* 36: 1843–1848, 1985.

37. THIBAULT, G., R. GARCIA, M. CANTIN, AND J. GENEST. Atrial natriuretic factor. Characterization and partial purification. *Hypertension Dallas* 5, Suppl. I: 75–80, 1983.

38. WILLIAMS, G. H., AND E. BRAUNWALD. Hypertensive vascular disease. In: *Harrison's Principles of Internal Medicine*, edited by R. G. Petersdorf, R. D. Adams, E. Braunwald, K. J. Isselbacher, J. B. Martin, and J. D. Wilson. New York: McGraw-Hill, 1983, vol. 10, p. 1475–1488.

39. YAMANAKA, M., B. GREENBERG, L. JOHNSON, J. SEILHAMER, M. BREWER, T. FRIEDEMANN, J. MILLER, S. ATLAS, J. LARAGH, J. LEWICKI, ET AL. Cloning and sequence analysis of the cDNA for the rat atrial natriuretic factor precursor. *Nature Lond.* 309: 719–722, 1984.

40. YANG-FENG, T. L., G. FLOYD-SMITH, M. NEMER, J. DROUIN, AND U. FRANKE. The pronatriodilatin gene is located on the distal short arm of human chromosome 1 and on mouse chromosome 4. *Am. J. Hum. Genet.* 37: 1117–1128, 1985.

41. ZIVIN, R. A., J. H. CONDRA, R. A. DIXON, N. G. SEIDAH, M. CHRÉTIEN, M. NEMER, M. CHAMBERLAND, AND J. DROUIN. Molecular cloning and characterization of DNA sequences encoding rat and human atrial natriuretic factors. *Proc. Natl. Acad. Sci. USA* 81: 6325–6329, 1984.

3

Mechanisms Controlling Release of Atrial Natriuretic Peptide

R. E. LANG, H. RUSKOAHO, M. TOTH, D. GANTEN,
T. UNGER, AND R. DIETZ

*German Institute for High Blood Pressure Research and Departments
of Pharmacology and Cardiology, University of Heidelberg,
Heidelberg, Federal Republic of Germany*

Intracellular Signals Mediating Atrial Natriuretic Peptide (ANP) Release
Humoral Factors in ANP Control
Nervous Control of ANP Release
Atrial Distension
Is ANP Release Controlled by Nervous Reflexes?
Conclusions

THE MYOENDOCRINE CELLS in the atria of the mammalian heart synthesize and secrete a hormone called atrial natriuretic peptide (ANP), which causes natriuresis and diuresis. Pharmacological studies in the isolated heart suggest that cytosolic calcium may regulate the release of ANP. The concentration of calcium in heart muscle cells depends on many factors, such as the action of humoral substances, cardiac nerve activity, heart rate, and resting length of the myocardial fibers. These factors may also contribute to the regulation of ANP secretion. The most important factor in the control of ANP release appears to be fiber length. Experimental and clinical observations indicate a direct correlation between secretion rate and atrial filling pressure. Little is known about the role of heart rate, autonomic nerve activity, and humoral factors in ANP regulation; further investigation is required.

The heart has always been considered critical in the mediation of volume-induced natriuresis and diuresis, since its low-pressure elements are able to sense the fullness of circulation. Recently, however, it was found that the heart is also the site where a natriuretic hormone is produced (4). This is not surprising, since it has long been speculated that another hormone is involved in the maintenance of salt-water homeostasis in addition to the renin-aldosterone system and vasopressin. This hormone, which is found in the atria but not the ventricles of the mammalian heart, is now known to be a peptide, whose synthesis closely resembles that of other peptide hormones (34). It is stored in the secretory granules of atrial myocytes and has been shown to be released in response to stimuli, which augment central blood volume (15, 43). Thus the heart is not only a pump but also acts to some extent like an endocrine gland.

In the past the mechanisms controlling hormone release have been the subject of intense research, and for most endocrine organs, hormone release is now relatively well understood. In principle, hormone secretion is regulated either by circulating factors or by autonomic nerves conveying information from a distant place, where the hormone's effects are sensed, to the gland. The release of ANP may be regulated similarly; however, the particular structure and functional duality of the myoendocrine cells, which are depolarized in regular intervals by electric pulses spreading through the atria, suggest that other mechanisms may be involved.

INTRACELLULAR SIGNALS MEDIATING ANP RELEASE

Much progress has been made during the past few years in elucidating how external signals are translated into internal signals that ultimately regulate a cellular process, such as secretion. Three internal signal pathways have been shown to be involved in the mediation of hormone release. One pathway employs the second-messenger cAMP, which is formed from ATP by the enzyme adenylate cyclase. A second pathway employs calcium ions, where cytosolic calcium may be increased by two mechanisms. The calcium can enter the cell through selective membrane channels or, more importantly, it can be mobilized from intracellular calcium pools, such as the sarcoplasmic reticulum. Release of calcium from intracellular stores is initiated by inosine 5'-triphosphate (ITP), which together with diacylglycerol (DAG) is generated from membrane phosphoinositides. Inosine 5'-triphosphate and DAG each represent one branch of the third pathway, the so-called phosphatidylinositol (PI) system. The final chemical step of all three signal pathways involves the phosphorylation of particular proteins, which may contribute to the transport and to the fusion of secretory granules with the cell membrane. This protein phosphorylation is mediated by protein kinases. The protein kinase activated by cAMP is called protein kinase A (3, 23). The so-called protein kinase C is activated by DAG. This activation requires the presence of calcium, which is mobilized from intracellular stores by ITP. Thus the two limbs of the PI system are synergistic in activating protein kinase C.

The contribution of each pathway to hormone secretion can be assessed with pharmacological agents that mimic the action of a particular second messenger. The calcium calmodulin pathway can be activated by the ionophore A23187 or the calcium channel agonist BAYK8644. Both A23187 and BAYK8644 introduce free calcium into the cell. Therefore they may also be used to mimic the action of ITP. Stimulation of protein kinase C can be achieved with certain phorbol esters, such as 12-O-tetradecaonylphorbol-13-acetate (TPA), which is structurally closely related to DAG. Finally, the cAMP pathway can be activated with forskolin, which stimulates adenylate cyclase (33).

We have studied the effects of these compounds on ANP release in the isolated perfused rat heart. The hearts were prepared according to the technique described by Langendorff (16). The aorta was cannulated superior to the aortic valve and perfused in a reversed direction with Krebs-Henseleit buffer. The coronary venous effluent was collected at 2-min intervals for determination of ANP by radioimmunoassay. The hearts were perfused for one hour to stabilize hormone-secretion rates. After a 10-min control period agonists were added to the perfusate, using an infusion rate of 0.5 ml/min for 30 min. Either ethanol or dimethyl sulfoxide (DMSO) was used as a vehicle at final concentrations <0.03%. Figure 1 shows that the vehicles alone did not influence the constant rate of ANP release. However, when a 5.7×10^{-7} M solution of calcium ionophore A23187 was added to the perfusion buffer, ANP secretion started to rise within ~5 min. The amount of ANP released reached a plateau after the next 5 min and remained at this level for the rest of the infusion.

To elucidate the role of protein kinase C in ANP liberation a number of phorbol esters were tested with respect to their effects on secretion of the hormone. As reported previously, a final concentration of 1.6×10^{-7} M phorbol-12,13-didecanoate (PDD) and TPA induced a slow developing release of ANP into the perfusate. Both compounds substitute for the natural biologically active protein kinase C activator DAG (23). The biologically nonactive phorbol ester 4α-phorbol-12,13-didecanoate (4αPDD) was infused into the hearts to test the specificity of these effects via the protein kinase C pathway. This phorbol ester did not significantly alter the basal secretion of ANP, compared with vehicle.

Because calcium and DAG act synergistically to activate protein kinase C it was anticipated that the combination of calcium ionophore plus TPA should result in a more-than-additive response. Indeed, when both substances were added simultaneously to the perfusion fluid, there was a much higher stimulation of ANP secretion than expected from the calculated additive value for these agents (29). This suggests that ANP secretion is a calcium-dependent process, as already shown for many other hormones (26, 28).

A role for calcium in the control of ANP secretion is further supported by another series of experiments, where the ionophore A23187 was substituted by the calcium channel agonist BAYK8644 for increasing cytosolic calcium concentration. At a dose of 4×10^{-7} M, BAYK8644 caused a gradual increase in ANP secretion to a maximum of ~200% of the basal secretion (Fig. 1). When given with TPA, there was a marked potentiation of the TPA-induced hormone secretion.

To explore the role of cAMP-dependent protein kinase in ANP secretion, forskolin was infused; forskolin is known to elevate cAMP levels in myocardium by activation of adenylate cyclase. Forskolin, at a concentration of 10^{-6} M in the perfusion fluid, induced a relatively small ANP release, which developed gradually, as observed with BAYK8644. Forskolin, in combination with TPA, also resulted in a potentiation of the phorbol ester effects (Fig. 1). The free cytosolic calcium may also play an important part in this process by linking the actions of the cAMP and PI pathway. It has been well established that in the heart a cAMP-dependent protein kinase catalyzes phosphorylation of sarcolemmal slow calcium channels. This increases the likelihood for

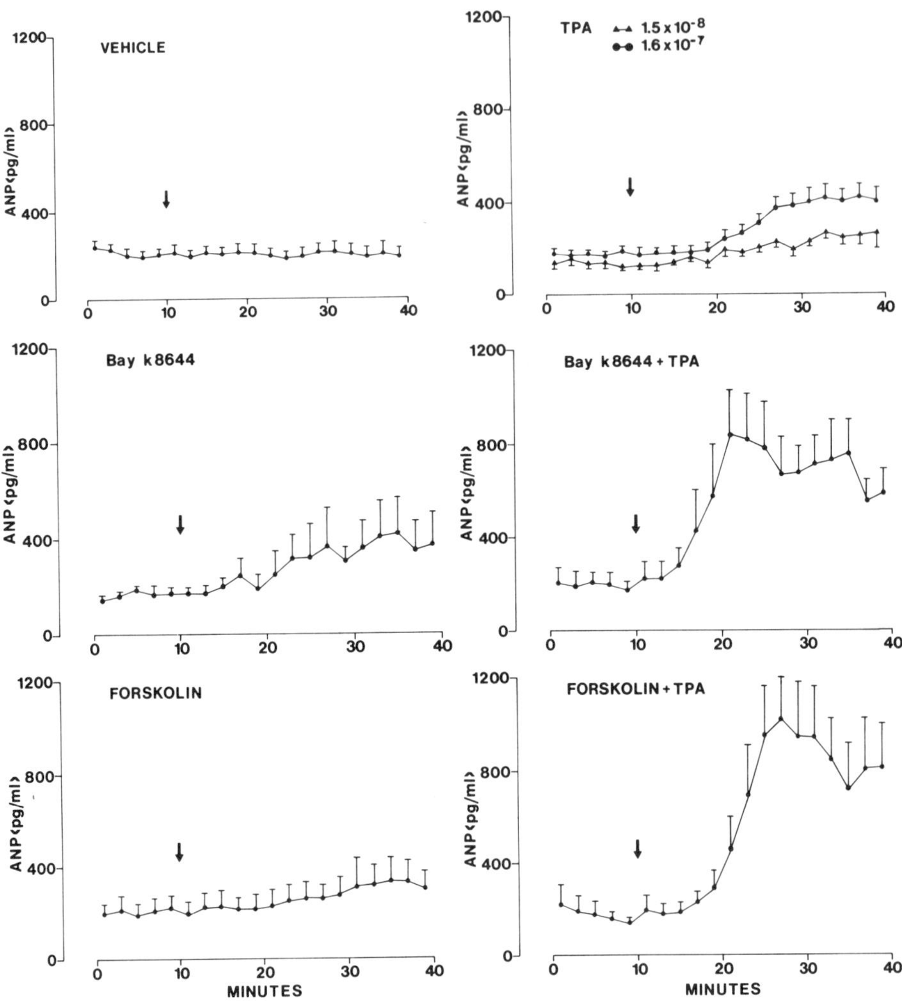

FIG. 1. Atrial natriuretic peptide (ANP) secretion into perfusate from isolated perfused rat hearts. Hearts were perfused (16) for 1 h with a constant flow of 5 ml/min to stabilize hormone-secretion rates. After 10-min control period, agonists were added (↓) to perfusion fluid with an infusion rate of 0.5 ml/min. Phorbolester was dissolved in dimethyl sulfoxide (DMSO), forskolin and the calcium channel agonist BAYK8644 were dissolved in ethanol, and all other substances were dissolved in Krebs-Henseleit solution. Final concentrations of DMSO and ethanol were <0.03%. Coronary venous effluents were collected at 2-min intervals and stored at −20°C until they were assayed for ANP-like immunoreactivity (ANPir) by radioimmunoassay. Vehicle group consisted of 4 infusions of DMSO, ethanol, and Krebs-Henseleit solution. The ANPir secretion is expressed as pg/ml perfusate; each point is the mean value ±SE for 5–12 separate experiments run on different isolated rat hearts. TPA, 12-O-tetradecanoylphorbol-13-acetate.

activation and enhances the influx of calcium into the myocyte (27). The elevated calcium may then contribute to the activation of protein kinase C. Thus, taken together, obviously the cytosolic calcium concentration is one of the most critical factors that determine ANP release. This is consistent with other observations made in many other endocrine systems, where the role of calcium, as a prerequisite for hormone secretion, has been recognized for many years (28).

If the factors regulating cytosolic free calcium in a particular endocrine cell are known, it should be possible to predict the mechanisms controlling hormone release from the gland. The ANP-synthesizing cells in the heart are specialized cardiocytes, which not only secrete a hormone but also show the basic properties of heart muscle cells, i.e., excitability, conductivity, and contractility. It can therefore be assumed that the cellular calcium in these cells is regulated in the same fashion as, for example, ventricular cardiocytes (35). The main factors determining the peak concentration of free calcium in a myocardial cell are known to be the amounts of calcium entering the cell through voltage-dependent calcium channels during depolarization and the release rate of calcium from the sarcoplasmic reticulum. Calcium influx is a function of the duration of action potential, the number of action potentials per unit time, and the number of activated calcium channels. All these parameters are mainly under the control of the autonomic nervous system, which may exert its action either directly on the cell through the release of neurotransmitters or indirectly by altering the heart rate. In addition, circulating substances such as epinephrine or glucagon could influence free cellular calcium concentration. The exact mechanism involved in the mobilization of calcium from the sarcoplasmic reticulum of cardiac cells is not completely understood; however, there is evidence that ITP is involved.

It has also been demonstrated that the cytosolic calcium concentration depends on the resting length of the myocardial fibers. Experiments with aequorin clearly show that calcium concentrations are increased by stretch and reduced after relaxation. This suggests that, in addition to heart rate and cardiac nerve activity, ANP secretion may be regulated by the tension of the atrial wall, which is a function of atrial filling pressure (1).

HUMORAL FACTORS IN ANP CONTROL

There is evidence that ANP release may be influenced by humoral factors acting directly on the heart. Sonnenberg et al. (37) and Sonnenberg and Veress (38) reported that incubation of isolated cardiac atria with epinephrine or arginine vasopressin results in an increased liberation of ANP. These authors concluded that the phosphatidylinositol phosphate system was involved in the mediation of these effects, because the response to epinephrine was attenuated in the presence of the α-adrenoceptor antagonist phentolamine and the vasopressin analogue dAVP was ineffective in contrast to arginine vasopressin. Intravenous administration of vasopressin, angiotensin II, or phenylephrine has recently been shown to increase plasma ANP levels in rats. This effect, however, is probably due to the vascular effects of these compounds, since the rise in ANP closely correlated with mean arterial pressure (22).

NERVOUS CONTROL OF ANP RELEASE

We have examined the effect of epinephrine on the release of ANP in the isolated perfused rat heart. Epinephrine was added to the perfusion fluid at a concentration of either 10^{-7} or 10^{-6} M. There was a dose-dependent rise in heart rate and force of contraction in association with a marked increase of ANP in the perfusate. The release of ANP was almost completely abolished by the β-adrenoceptor antagonist propranolol. On the other hand, ANP release was also stimulated by addition of 10^{-6} M methoxamine, an α_1-adrenoceptor agonist. Thus both β- and α-adrenoceptors appear to mediate the epinephrine effect on ANP release.

Acetylcholine also stimulates ANP release from isolated rat atria in vitro (38). We found that perfusion of the isolated heart with 10^{-5} or 10^{-6} M acetylcholine resulted in a short rise in hormone release followed by a gradual decline. The rise in ANP was blocked by atropine, suggesting involvement of a muscarinic receptor.

The observation that both acetylcholine and catecholamines alter the ANP-secretion rate implies that autonomic nerves participate in the regulation of this hormone. Recently Ledsome and co-workers (20) addressed this question in studies in the dog. They observed that electrical stimulation of the right ansa subclavia did not change plasma ANP levels, although heart rate increased by 100 beats/min. This is somewhat surprising, because other studies show that ANP secretion is dependent on the rate of depolarization. Schiebinger and Linden (31) recently demonstrated that when the isolated left rat atrium was paced at 3 Hz the release of ANP was more than doubled. Secretion was also enhanced when atrial tension was increased. The authors concluded that the rate of contractions, in addition to atrial tension, determines hormone release.

Clinical studies provide evidence that heart rate can control ANP secretion. Several groups have reported that plasma ANP levels are elevated during tachycardia or atrial pacing at high frequencies (42). It is, however, difficult to decide whether increased heart rate or atrial tension is responsible for the increased hormone secretion, since atrial filling pressure may increase under these circumstances.

ATRIAL DISTENSION

The most effective and best documented stimulus for ANP release appears to be atrial distension. The idea of a natriuretic hormone released in response to stretch is very old. As early as 1956, Henry, Gauer, and Reeves (9) demonstrated that inflation of a balloon in the left atrium resulted in a marked rise in urine flow. Henry and Pearce (10) postulated that this diuresis was due to the reflex inhibition of the release of antidiuretic hormone, which depended on stimulation of left atrial receptors and increased afferent impulses in the vagus. Suppression of antidiuretic hormone secretion, however, could not

entirely explain the increase in urine output observed during left atrial distension, since a diuretic response was still obtained in the presence of exogenous
antidiuretic hormone and was associated with increases in sodium excretion
(18). Baisset et al. (2) demonstrated that balloon distension of the right atrium
in dogs resulted in increased urine flow and sodium excretion. Plasma vasopressin levels were not affected by this stimulus (4). These studies suggested
that the renal response to atrial distension is mediated by at least two
mechanisms. One mechanism regulates diuresis through vasopressin; a second
controls both natriuresis and diuresis through a humoral factor, now known
to be ANP.

Dietz (7) first demonstrated in an isolated heart-lung preparation that
atrial stretch results in the release of natriuretic factor directly from the heart.
Right atrial pressure was varied by increasing venous return. The perfusate
collected at high atrial pressure produced a significant diuresis and natriuresis
when infused into rats.

Using a similar preparation, we found that the release of ANP-like
immunoreactive material is closely correlated to right atrial pressure. These
experiments were carried out in isolated perfused rat hearts, which were
perfused through the aorta with Krebs-Ringer solution at constant flow. The
upper vena cava was also cannulated and buffer was infused into the right
atrium. Increasing the infusion rate produced a rise in right atrial pressure,
which was continuously monitored by a pressure transducer connected to a
catheter that was inserted into the lower vena cava. The perfusate was collected
from a cannula inserted into the pulmonary artery and ANP concentration
was determined by radioimmunoassay.

A typical response to volume loading in an isolated perfused heart is
shown in Figure 2. The increase in total flow from 7.5 ml/min during the
control period to 9.8 ml/min during the stimulation period produced a rapid
increase in right atrial pressure. Heart rate and force of contraction showed a
slight decrease. There was a linear correlation ($P < 0.001$) between the rise in
right atrial pressure and the release of ANP, indicating that muscle length
determines the rate of ANP secretion (Fig. 3).

The material released before and during atrial distension was characterized by high-performance liquid chromatography. It was found to elute as a
single peak at the position of synthetic Ile[12]-ANP, which appears to be the
major circulating form of ANP in the rat (32, 40).

Atrial stretch has also been reported to provoke ANP release in vivo.
Ledsome et al. (19) showed that mitral obstruction increased plasma ANP in
dogs. In contrast, pulmonary vein distension, which is known to cause suppression of arginine vasopressin, did not affect ANP levels (19, 20). Distension
of the atrial wall is a function of atrial filling pressure, which can be experi-
mentally manipulated in many ways. The procedure most frequently used in
recent studies of ANP release is to increase the extracellular fluid volume by
intravenous infusion of saline or blood.

We have previously shown that volume loading stimulates ANP release
in the rat (14). Rats in which catheters had been inserted into the femoral

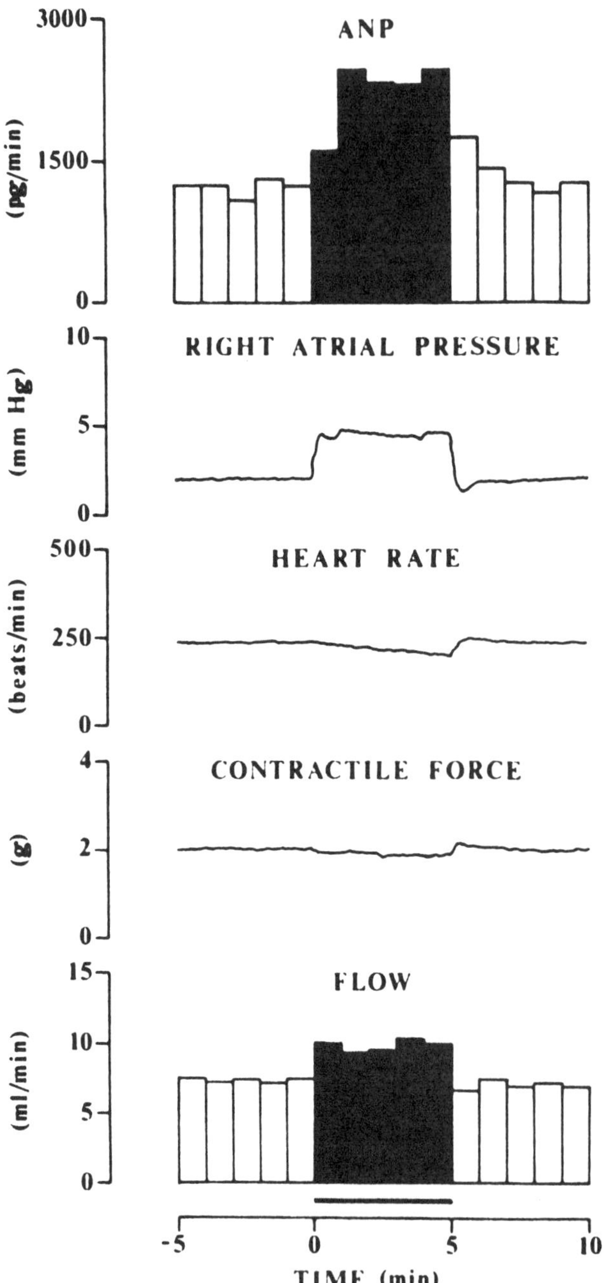

FIG. 2. Response to volume loading of right atrium in one isolated perfused rat heart. ANP, ANF-like immunoreactive material (ANF, atrial natriuretic factor). Flow, coronary flow plus additional perfusion during stimulation. Perfusate was collected over 1-min periods. —, Duration of volume loading.

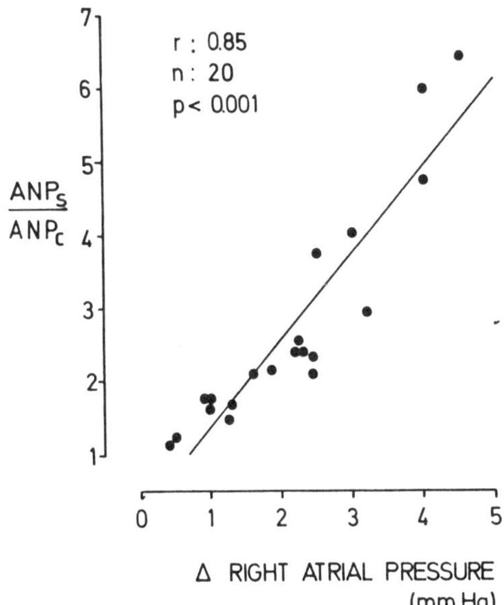

FIG. 3. Relationship between changes in rate of ANP release and right atrial pressure in isolated perfused rat hearts. ANP_s/ANP_c, ratio between maximal rate of ANP release during distension and mean control value. ●, Value of one distension experiment. Regression equation for ANP_s/ANP_c (Y) against Δ right atrial pressure (X) was Y = 77.85 ± 119.06 X.

vein were divided into three groups. One group served as a control; the other two received either a 2-ml or 8-ml saline infusion, which corresponds to a 7 or 30% volume expansion, respectively. Changes in right atrial pressure during volume loading were measured by means of a catheter inserted into the right atrium through the jugular vein. There was a rapid volume-dependent increase in right atrial pressure, which was accompanied by a transient rise in plasma ANP concentration.

Acute infusion of a saline load has also been shown to increase plasma ANP levels in humans (30, 43). Long-term alterations in blood volume may also be produced by changes in dietary sodium intake. Tanaka et al. (39) were the first to demonstrate that high-salt intake results in an increase in circulating ANP in rats. Similar observations were recently made in humans (30, 36).

Right atrial pressure is also altered by changes in posture, which affect venous return. There are some studies that report that head-down tilt causes plasma ANP levels to rise. In these studies, hormone levels doubled during 20° head-down tilt and increased almost threefold after 5 min in upside-down position (11, 17).

Another maneuver causing central hypervolemia is head-out water immersion. This procedure induces a significant diuresis and natriuresis without any alteration in glomerular filtration rate or renal blood flow. As recently demonstrated in anesthetized rats, vertical immersion in warm water results in a pronounced increase in plasma ANP, which is directly correlated with the elevation in right atrial pressure (12). Plasma ANP was reported to rise similarly in humans within the first 30 min during head-out total-body water immersion (24).

Atrial stretch appears to be an important mechanism in controlling ANP release. Studies have demonstrated that ANP plasma concentrations are elevated in pathological states associated with increased atrial filling pressure, such as cardiac disease, renal failure with fluid retention, pulmonary diseases, and primary aldosteronism. Tikkanen et al. (41) demonstrated that ANP is increased in plasma of patients with congestive heart failure. Our group has reported that ANP is high in plasma of children with congenital heart diseases and bronchopulmonary dysplasia (15). We have also found that plasma ANP levels are significantly correlated with atrial filling pressure in patients who underwent cardiac catheterization. This confirms our earlier studies with the isolated perfused rat heart. As shown in Figure 4, there is a positive correlation between plasma ANP and right atrial pressure in patients with mitral stenosis. The correlation is observed for many other valvular heart diseases and for cardiomyopathy (13).

Renal failure is another disease where atrial filling pressure can be increased due to fluid retention. We have studied plasma ANP in patients with end-stage renal failure and found markedly elevated levels, as compared with healthy controls and patients with less severe impairment of renal function (25). The hormone concentration dropped significantly after hemodialysis. This decline was probably due to the reduction in extracellular fluid volume, because it correlated strongly with the loss in body weight after hemodialysis.

IS ANP RELEASE CONTROLLED BY NERVOUS REFLEXES?

The atria of the heart contain numerous unencapsulated nerve endings, which histologically resemble arterial baroreceptors and are believed to monitor the volume of blood (8, 21). An increase in central blood volume raises the pressure within the atria and activates these volume receptors. Nerve impulses arising from these receptors traveling via the vagus nerves to the brain may alter vasopressin secretion and sympathetic nerve activity and thereby in part contribute to the renal responses observed during atrial distension. There is little evidence that the release of ANP depends on a reflex involving atrial receptors. Ledsome et al. (19, 20) have reported that in the dog the increase in plasma ANP after mitral obstruction was not affected by bilateral cervical vagotomy or cardiac β-adrenoceptor blockade. Similarly, Katsube et al. (12) found that the pronounced rise in ANP measured in rats during water immersion was not prevented by bilateral transection of the vagi. This is consistent with the view that ANP secretion from the heart is stimulated directly by stretch of the atrial wall.

CONCLUSIONS

The best documented and probably most important stimulus of ANP release is atrial stretch. Secretion of ANP may be triggered directly by the rise

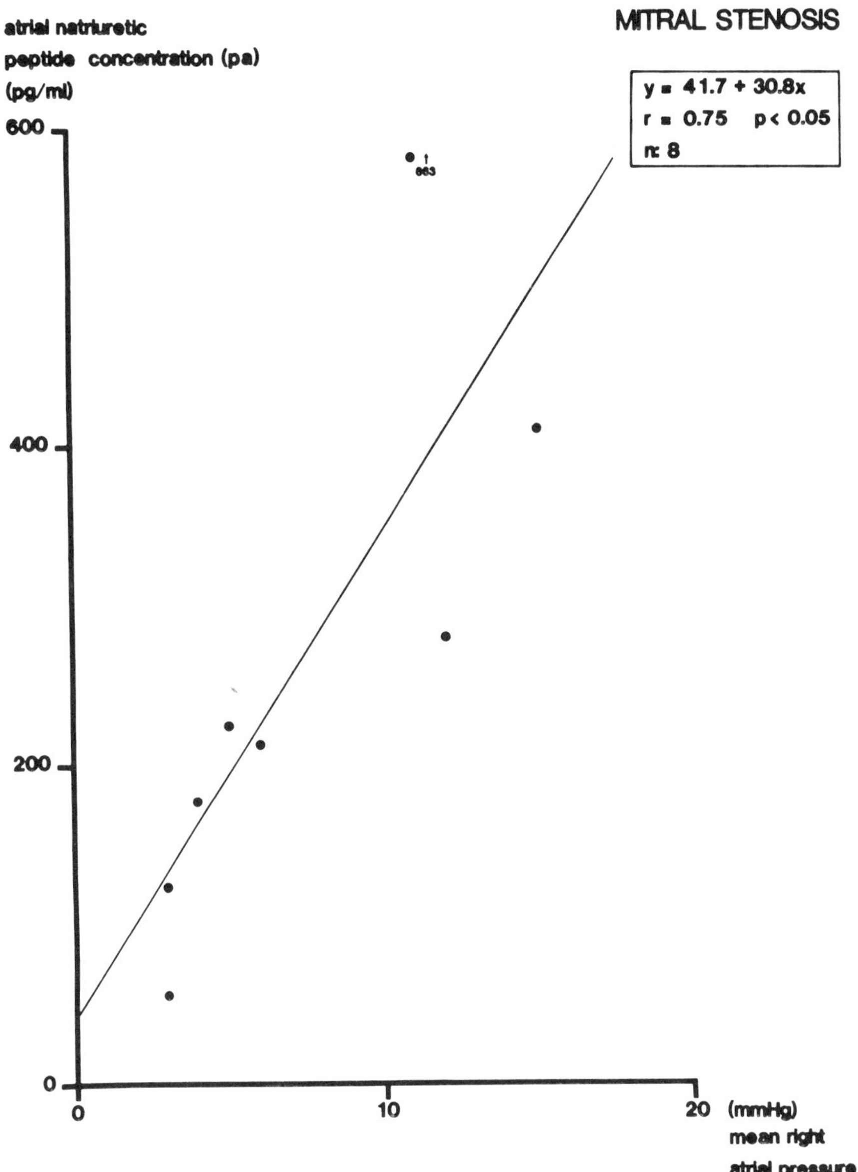

FIG. 4. Relationship between right atrial filling pressure (abscissa) and plasma concentration of ANP (ordinate) in patients with mitral stenosis.

in free intracellular calcium, which is observed when the resting length of myocardial fibers is increased. The role of the other intracellular signals in this process is not completely understood. There is some controversy over whether the heart rate influences ANP secretion. In vitro experiments demonstrate that in addition to tension the rate of contraction plays some part, but the results obtained from in vivo studies are not conclusive. Neurotransmitters alter the rate of ANP release, probably by mediation of the cAMP and PI system. This is indirect evidence for a role of autonomic nerves in the control of ANP release. Although stretch-induced ANP secretion does not require an intact innervation of the heart, this does not necessarily exclude a modulatory effect of the nervous system. There is little evidence that humoral factors directly influence ANP release, but epinephrine may have some effect.

REFERENCES

1. ALLEN, D. G., AND S. KURIHARA. The effects of muscle length on intracellular calcium transients in mammalian cardiac muscle. *J. Physiol. Lond.* 327: 79–94, 1971.
2. BAISSET, A. E., L. DOUSTE-BLAZY, AND P. MONTASTRUC. Reduction de la secretion d'aldosterone sous l'effect d'une distension auriculaire. *J. Physiol. Paris* 51: 393–396, 1959.
3. BERRIDGE, M. J. Inositol trisphosphate and diacylglycerol as second messengers. *Biochem. J.* 220: 345–360, 1984.
4. BRENNAN, L. A., JR., R. L. MALVIN, K. E. JOCHIM, AND D. E. ROBERTS. Influence of right and left atrial receptors on plasma concentrations of ADH and renin. *Am. J. Physiol.* 221: 273–278, 1971.
5. CANTIN, M., AND J. GENEST. The heart and the atrial natriuretic factor. *Endocr. Rev.* 6: 107–127, 1985.
6. DE BOLD, A. J., H. B. BORENSTEIN, A. T. VERESS, AND H. SONNENBERG. A rapid and potent natriuretic response to intravenous injection of atrial myocardial extract in rats. *Life Sci.* 28: 89–94, 1981.
7. DIETZ, J. R. Release of natriuretic factor from rat heart-lung preparation by atrial distension. *Am. J. Physiol.* 247 (*Regulatory Integrative Comp. Physiol.* 16): R1093–R1096, 1984.
8. GOETZ, K. L., G. C. BOND, AND D. D. BLOXHAM. Atrial receptors and renal function. *Physiol. Rev.* 55: 157–205, 1975.
9. HENRY, J. P., O. H. GAUER, AND J. L. REEVES. Evidence of the atrial location of receptors influencing urine flow. *Circ. Res.* 4: 85–90, 1956.
10. HENRY, J. P., AND J. W. PEARCE. The possible role of cardiac atrial stress receptors in the induction of changes in urine flow. *J. Physiol. Lond.* 131: 572–585, 1956.
11. HODSMAN, G. P., K. TSUNODA, K. OGAWA, AND C. I. JOHNSTON. Effects of posture on circulating atrial natriuretic peptide. *Lancet* 2: 1427, 1985.
12. KATSUBE, N., D. SCHWARTZ, AND P. NEEDLEMAN. Release of atriopeptin in the rat by vasoconstrictors or water immersion correlates with changes in right atrial pressure. *Biochem. Biophys. Res. Commun.* 133: 937–944, 1985.
13. LANG, R. E., R. DIETZ, A. MERKEL, H. RUSKOAHO, D. GANTEN, AND T. UNGER. Plasma atrial natriuretic peptide (ANP) values in cardiac disease. *J. Hypertens.* 4, Suppl. 2: 119–123, 1986.
14. LANG, R. E., H. THOELKEN, D. GANTEN, F. C. LUFT, H. RUSKOAHO, AND T. UNGER. Atrial natriuretic factor—a circulating hormone stimulated by volume loading. *Nature Lond.* 314: 264–266, 1985.
15. LANG, R. E., T. UNGER, D. GANTEN, J. WEIL, F. BIDLINGMAIER, AND D. DOHLEMANN. Atrial natriuretic peptide concentrations in plasma of children with congenital heart and pulmonary diseases. *Br. Med. J.* 291: 1241, 1985.
16. LANGENDORFF, O. Untersuchungen am überlebenden Sägetierherzen. *Pfluegers Arch.* 61: 291–332, 1985.
17. LAROSE, P., S. MELOCHE, P. DU SOUICH, A. DELÉAN, AND H. ONG. Radioimmunoassay of atrial natriuretic factor: human plasma levels. *Biochem. Biophys. Res. Commun.* 130: 553–558, 1985.
18. LEDSOME, J. R., R. J. LINDEN, AND W. J. O'CONNOR. The mechanisms by which distension of the left atrium produces diuresis in anesthetized dogs. *J. Physiol. Lond.* 159: 87–100, 1961.
19. LEDSOME, J. R., N. WILSON, C. A. COURNEYA, AND A. J. RANKIN. Release of atrial natriuretic peptide by atrial distension. *Can. J. Physiol. Pharmacol.* 63: 739–742, 1985.
20. LEDSOME, J. R., N. WILSON, A. J. RANKIN, AND C. A. COURNEYA. Mechanism of release of atrial natriuretic peptide (ANP) (abstr.). *Federation Proc.* 44: 7706, 1985.
21. LINDEN, R. J. Atrial reflexes and renal function. *Am. J. Cardiol.* 44: 879–883, 1979.

22. MANNING, P. T., D. SCHWARTZ, N. C. KATSUBE, S. W. HOLMBERG, AND P. NEEDLEMAN. Vasopressin-stimulated release of atriopeptin: endocrine antagonists in fluid homeostasis. *Science Wash. DC* 229: 395–397, 1985.
23. NISHIZUKA, Y., Y. TAKAI, A. KISHIMOTO, U. KIKKAWA, AND K. KAIBUCHI. Phospholipid turnover in hormone action. *Recent Prog. Horm. Res.* 40: 301–344, 1984.
24. OGIHARA, T., J. KAWASAKI, Y. TABUCHI, K. HASHIZUME, Y. KUMAHARA, K. KANGAWA, AND H. MATSUO. Changes in plasma atrial natriuretic polypeptide (ANP) concentration during head-out water immersion and saline infusion in normal man (abstr.). *Hypertension Dallas* 7: 838, 1985.
25. RASCHER, W., T. TULASSAY, AND R. E. LANG. Atrial natriuretic peptide in plasma of volume-overloaded children with chronic renal failure. *Lancet* 2: 303–305, 1985.
26. RASMUSSEN, H. Cellular calcium metabolism. *Ann. Intern. Med.* 98: 809–816, 1983.
27. REUTER, H. Calcium channel modulation by neurotransmitters, enzymes and drugs. *Nature Lond.* 301: 569–574, 1983.
28. RUBIN, R. P. Stimulus-secretion coupling. In: *Cell Biology of the Secretory Process*, edited by M. Cantin. Basel: Karger, 1984, p. 52–72.
29. RUSKOAHO, H., M. TOTH, AND R. E. LANG. Atrial natriuretic peptide secretion: synergistic effect of phorbolester and A23187. *Biochem. Biophys. Res. Commun.* 133: 581–588, 1985.
30. SAGNELLA, G. A., A. C. SHORE, N. D. MARKANDU, AND G. A. MACGREGOR. Effects of changes in dietary sodium intake and saline infusion on immunoreactive atrial natriuretic peptide in human plasma. *Lancet* 2: 1208–1211, 1985.
31. SCHIEBINGER, R. J., AND J. M. LINDEN. The influence of stretch and rate of contraction on ANF secretion by rat atria in vitro (abstr.). *Hypertension Dallas* 7: 846, 1985.
32. SCHWARTZ, D., M. GELLER, P. T. MANNING, N. R. SIEGEL, K. F. FOK, C. E. SMITH, AND P. NEEDLEMAN. Ser-Leu-Arg-Arg-atriopeptin III: the major circulating form of atrial peptide. *Science Wash. DC* 229: 397–400, 1985.
33. SEAMON, K. B., W. PADGETT, AND J. W. DALY. Forskolin: unique diterpene activator of adenylate cyclase in membranes and in intact cells. *Proc. Natl. Acad. Sci. USA* 78: 3363–3367, 1981.
34. SEIDMAN, C. E., K. D. BLOCH, J. ZISFEIN, J. A. SMITH, E. HABER, C. HOMCY, A. D. DUBY, E. CHOI, R. M. GRAHAM, AND J. G. SEIDMAN. Molecular studies of the atrial natriuretic factor gene. *Hypertension Dallas* 7, Suppl. I: 131–134, 1985.
35. SHAMOO, A. E., AND I. S. AMBUDKAR. Regulation of calcium transport in cardiac cells. *Can. J. Physiol. Pharmacol.* 62: 9–22, 1984.
36. SHENKER, Y., R. S. SIDER, E. A. OSTAFIN, AND R. J. GREKIN. Plasma levels of immunoreactive atrial natriuretic factor in healthy subjects and in patients with edema. *J. Clin. Invest.* 76: 1684–1687, 1985.
37. SONNENBERG, H., R. F. KREBS, AND A. T. VERESS. Release of atrial natriuretic factor from incubated rat heart atria. *IRCS Med. Sci. Libr. Compend.* 12: 783–784, 1984.
38. SONNENBERG, H., AND A. T. VERESS. Cellular mechanism of release of atrial natriuretic factor. *Biochem. Biophys. Res. Commun.* 124: 443–449, 1984.
39. TANAKA, I., K. S. MISONO, AND T. INAGAMI. Atrial natriuretic factor in rat hypothalamus, atria and plasma: determination by specific radioimmunoassay. *Biochem. Biophys. Res. Commun.* 124: 663–668, 1984.
40. THIBAULT, G., C. LAZURE, E. L. SCHIFFRIN, J. GUTKOWSKA, L. CHARTIER, R. GARCIA, N. G. SEIDAH, M. CHRÉTIEN, J. GENEST, AND M. CANTIN. Identification of a biologically active circulating form of rat atrial natriuretic factor. *Biochem. Biophys. Res. Commun.* 130: 981–986, 1985.
41. TIKKANEN, I., F. FYHRQUIST, K. METSÄRINNE, AND R. LEIDENIUS. Plasma atrial natriuretic peptide in cardiac disease and during infusion in healthy volunteers. *Lancet* 2: 66–69, 1985.
42. TIKKANEN, I., K. METSÄRINNE, AND F. FYHRQUIST. Atrial natriuretic peptide in paroxysmal supraventricular tachycardia (letter). *Lancet* 2: 40–41, 1985.
43. YAMAIJ, T., M. ISHIBASHI, AND F. TAKAKU. Atrial natriuretic factor in human blood. *J. Clin. Invest.* 76: 1705–1709, 1985.

4

Atriopeptin Expression in the Ventricle

ROGER C. WIEGAND, MARK L. DAY, CHARLES P. RODI,
DAVID SCHWARTZ, AND PHILIP NEEDLEMAN

*Department of Biological Sciences, Monsanto Company, Chesterfield, Missouri;
and Department of Pharmacology, Washington University
Medical School, St. Louis, Missouri*

Ventricular Hypertrophy
Dexamethasone Treatment
Dexamethasone and Hypertrophy Give an Additive Effect
Form of the Accumulated Material
Dexamethasone Affects Heart Cells Directly
Atriopeptin Expression in Ventricles During Development

ATRIOPEPTINS COMPRISE A FAMILY of small peptides, originally isolated from rat atria, that exert potent effects on natriuresis, diuresis, and vascular smooth muscle relaxation (3, 5, 17). The active peptides range from 21 to 33 amino acids in length and differ only in the number of residues flanking a 17–amino acid disulfide-linked core. A 126–amino acid prohormone is stored in granules in both atria and is released from heart cells in culture (2). After pharmacological stimulation or atrial stretch, atriopeptin (AP) is found in the circulation primarily as the 28–amino acid peptide, AP28 (10, 24).

Levels of AP and of AP mRNA can be affected by chronic manipulation of dietary salt and water intake (15, 23). In water-deprived animals, AP immunoreactive material (APir) is increased in the atria while AP mRNA levels are decreased. In contrast, a high-salt diet results in decreased APir and increased AP mRNA levels in the atria. In these cases, as well as in the short-term release induced by 1-deamino-Arg^8-vasopressin (12), plasma levels of APir are inversely related to atrial content.

Atriopeptin has been demonstrated at low levels in a variety of nonatrial tissues (6, 13, 14, 18, 22), but AP mRNA has been reported only in the atrium and ventricle (25). In other tissues the levels of AP observed are generally consistent with AP being bound to the receptors in the tissue (1, 16). The ventricle has much higher levels of AP and has very low levels of AP receptor. The peptide concentration in the adult ventricle, ~300-fold lower than in atria, is thus likely to result from synthesis rather than binding to AP receptors.

VENTRICULAR HYPERTROPHY

Ventricular hypertrophy, produced by constriction of the abdominal aorta, has been shown to result in the appearance of electron-dense, membrane-

33

bound granules in the ventricular myocytes that are similar in structure to the AP-containing atrial granules (7). Based on this observation, the AP content of normal and hypertrophied ventricles was examined. Stored APir levels were found to be elevated about threefold over sham-operated controls in the left but not right ventricle (Fig. 1). In the same animals the levels of AP mRNA were also determined and found to be increased by a similar amount (Fig. 2). At the same time, left atrial APir content is depressed and circulating APir is somewhat increased. The effect on AP mRNA is at least somewhat specific. Although one of the effects of hypertrophy is an increase in the general level of protein synthesis, the relative levels of mRNA for creatine kinase (CK) are unchanged during treatment. Creatine kinase is made throughout cardiac muscle and is not known to be regulated.

DEXAMETHASONE TREATMENT

Dexamethasone is a synthetic glucocorticoid that has been shown to affect the regulation of a wide variety of genes. The human gene encoding AP contains a sequence in its second intron that has been reported to be similar to a consensus glucocorticoid receptor–binding site (20). There is no obvious

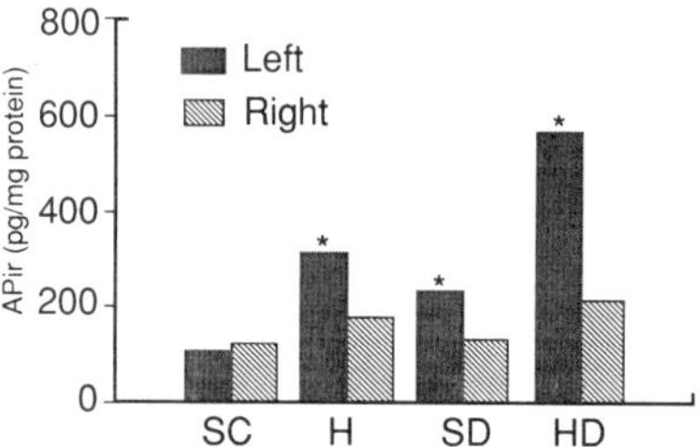

FIG. 1. Atriopeptin immunoreactive material (APir) in left and right ventricle; APir was measured in acid extracts of left and right ventricles of rats after no treatment (SC, sham-operated control), left ventricular hypertrophy (H), dexamethasone treatment (SD, sham-operated, dexamethasone-treated), and combined treatments (HD, left ventricular hypertrophy, dexamethasone-treated). *Significantly different ($P < 0.05$) from the sham-operated control.

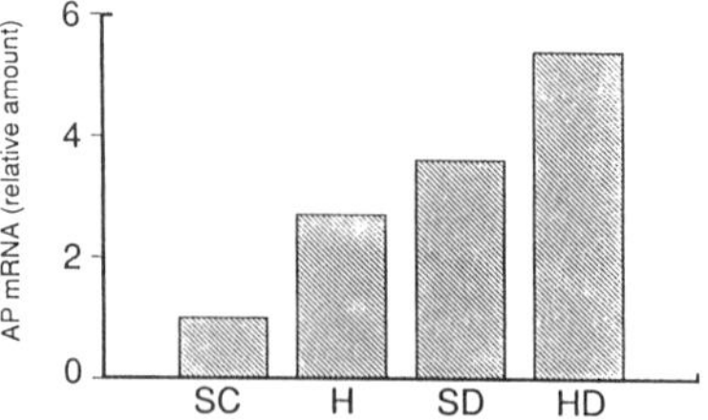

FIG. 2. Accumulation of AP mRNA in left ventricle. The AP mRNA was measured by quantitative Northern blotting in left ventricles of rats after no treatment (SC, sham-operated control), left ventricular hypertrophy (H), dexamethasone treatment (SD, sham-operated, dexamethasone-treated), and combined treatments (HD, left ventricular hypertrophy, dexamethasone-treated). Figure shows mean increase in AP mRNA relative to sham-operated control. Data are taken from many separate experiments; each experiment showed significant ($P < 0.05$) increases in AP mRNA for hypertrophy, dexamethasone, or the combined treatments.

similarity to reported consensus glucocorticoid receptor–binding sequences in the rat gene. However, functional receptor-binding sequences vary widely and may be present nonetheless. Indeed, both stored APir and accumulated AP mRNA increase in the left ventricle of rats in response to treatment with 2.5 mg/kg dexamethasone administered intraperitoneally at 48 and 24 h prior to killing (Figs. 1 and 2). These levels of dexamethasone have a substantial effect on the animals, including an overall body weight loss of 20–30%. The weight of the heart is unaffected by this treatment (9). The mRNA levels for CK are unchanged by treatment with dexamethasone, indicating that there is specificity of the effect and not simply an overall increase in the synthetic ability of the heart. Plasma APir is decreased by treatment with dexamethasone, and atrial levels are essentially unchanged. Neither stored APir nor AP mRNA levels are affected by dexamethasone in the right ventricle. Unlike hypertrophy, which specifically affects the left side, dexamethasone was expected to exert a similar effect on both ventricles. Both the left and right ventricles have receptors for dexamethasone (21). This unexpected specificity may reflect some fundamental difference in the roles or functioning of the left and right ventricles.

DEXAMETHASONE AND HYPERTROPHY GIVE AN ADDITIVE EFFECT

The administration of dexamethasone to animals with hypertrophied left ventricles results in increases in both protein and mRNA that are greater than those seen for either treatment alone (Figs. 1 and 2). Because of the difficulty of establishing a dose-response relationship for hypertrophy, it is not possible

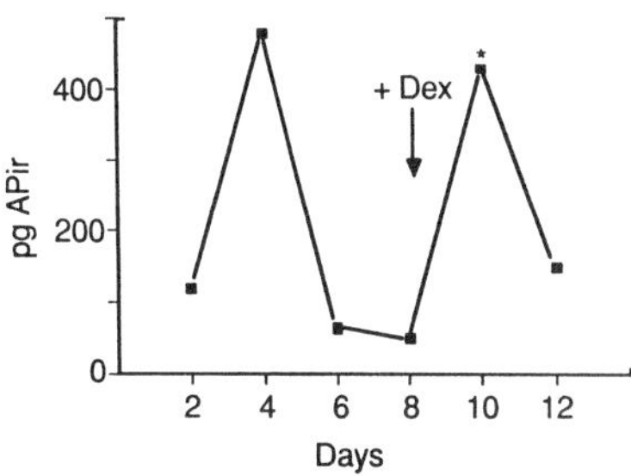

FIG. 3. Release of immunoreactive AP (APir) from cultured cardiocytes after addition of dexamethasone. Primary cultures of cardiocytes in serum-free media undergo a spontaneous release of APir, which subsides after 6 days in culture. Addition of dexamethasone at day 8 results in a substantial additional release of APir into the medium. *Significantly higher ($P < 0.01$) than the untreated control.

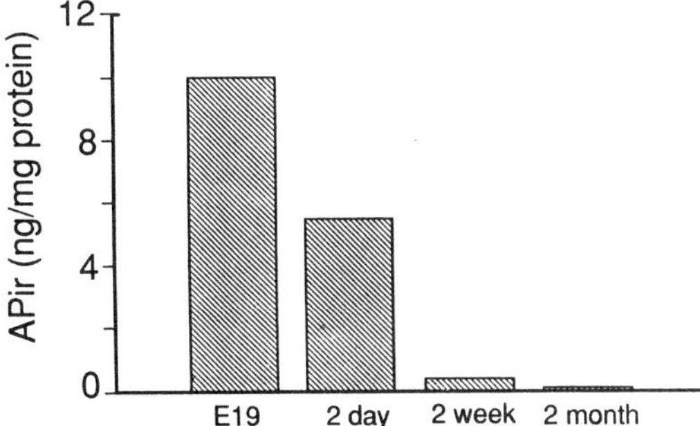

FIG. 4. Ventricular AP declines rapidly with age. Whole lower hearts were taken from rats at embryonic stage E19 and at the indicated times postnatally. Immunoreactive AP (APir) was measured by radioimmunoassay in acid-soluble extracts of the material. Values for E19 and 2 day are significantly higher ($P < 0.05$) than at 2 wk or 2 mo.

to determine whether this additivity reflects increases due to different mechanisms or simply submaximal stimulation of the same mechanism. The total amount of AP mRNA in the ventricle is substantial. Correcting for the difference in tissue mass, ventricular AP mRNA accounts for about one-third of the AP mRNA in the hearts of dexamethasone-treated, hypertrophied animals.

FORM OF THE ACCUMULATED MATERIAL

The AP mRNA accumulated in the ventricle in response to dexamethasone, hypertrophy, or the combined treatment appears to be identical to the mRNA normally made in the atria. The length of the mRNA is the same on Northern blot analysis and the 5′ end of the mRNA is identical, as judged by primer extension. The stored form of the protein is also identical in atria and ventricles. In both tissues, AP is stored as the 126–amino acid prohormone. Atriopeptin isolated from other nonatrial sources, such as the hypothalamus, eye, or kidney, is present in a low-molecular-weight form (6, 13, 14, 18, 22). The low-molecular-weight AP found in these tissues is in very low abundance and may represent AP bound to receptors. Cardiac myocytes lack AP receptors (1), and the amount of AP present is far in excess of the amount that might be accounted for by blood contamination. If this is coupled with the presence of atrial-like granules and AP mRNA that is engaged on polysomes (E. Tolunay, unpublished observations), there can be little doubt that AP is being synthesized in the ventricular tissue.

DEXAMETHASONE AFFECTS HEART CELLS DIRECTLY

Dexamethasone has many effects on a treated animal. A priori it is not possible to determine whether any given effect is the result of the direct action of the drug or a reaction to one of the actions of the drug. The direct effect of dexamethasone treatment on AP has been demonstrated with ventricular cells in culture. On being placed in culture, cells from the ventricles of two-day-old rats undergo a spontaneous release of APir. After the AP release has returned to base line a second release can be induced by addition of dexamethasone to the culture medium (Fig. 3; C. P. Rodi, unpublished observations). The effect of dexamethasone therefore need not be mediated through any other part of the body.

ATRIOPEPTIN EXPRESSION IN VENTRICLES DURING DEVELOPMENT

The observation of the spontaneous release of APir from ventricular cells in culture led to an examination of the expression of AP in very young animals. As shown in Figure 4, APir levels decline dramatically between birth and 2 mo postnatal in the rat. At the same time the AP mRNA levels in the ventricle decrease similarly (M. L. Day and C. P. Rodi, unpublished observations). In the neonate the AP mRNA concentrations are about the same in atria and in ventricles. By 2 mo the differential is ~100:1.

In ventricular hypertrophy the heart cells have been described as reverting to a fetal-like state (7). This structural resemblance apparently extends to including the expression of the AP gene. The AP gene is normally expressed at a very high level [0.5–1% of poly(A)$^+$ RNA] in adult atrial tissue (15) and at a moderate level [0.01% of poly(A)$^+$ RNA] in adult ventricle. In the neonate the AP mRNA concentration is 10–20 times that of the adult or 0.1–0.2% of the poly(A)$^+$ RNA. Consistent with this, membrane-bound electron-dense granules appear in the atria and ventricles of embryonic humans, mice, and rats (4, 11). These granules then disappear in later embryonic life from the ventricle but remain in the atrium. Atriopeptin has been demonstrated to have mitogenic activity on one cell type, adrenal zona glomerulosa (8), and given the timing of AP appearance in the ventricle, AP may have a role in the normal growth and development of the heart.

REFERENCES

1. BIANCHI, C., J. GUTKOWSKA, G. THIBAULT, R. GARCIA, J. GENEST, AND M. CANTIN. Radioautographic localization of ^{125}I-atrial natriuretic factor (ANF) in rat tissues. *Histochemistry* 82: 441–452, 1985.
2. BLOCH, K. D., J. A. SCOTT, J. B. ZISFEIN, J. T. FALLON, M. N. MARGOLIES, C. E. SEIDMAN, G. R. MATSUEDA, C. J. HOMCY, R. M. GRAHAM, AND J. G. SEIDMAN. Biosynthesis and secretion of proatrial natriuretic factor by cultured rat cardiocytes. *Science Wash. DC* 230: 1168–1171, 1985.
3. CANTIN, M., AND J. GENEST. The heart and the atrial natriuretic factor. *Endocr. Rev.* 6: 107–127, 1985.
4. CHALLICE, C. E., AND S. VIRÁGH. The embryologic development of the mammalian heart. In: *Ultrastructure of the Mammalian Heart*, edited by C. E. Challice and S. Virágh. New York: Academic, 1973, p. 91–126.
5. DE BOLD, A. J. Atrial natriuretic factor: a hormone produced by the heart. *Science Wash. DC* 230: 767–769, 1985.
6. GLEMBOTSKI, C. C., G. M. WILDEY, AND T. R. GIBSON. Molecular forms of immunoactive atrial natriuretic peptide in the rat hypothalamus and atrium. *Biochem. Biophys. Res. Commun.* 129: 671–678, 1985.
7. HATT, P.-Y. Cellular changes and damage in mechanically overloaded hearts. In: *Recent Advances in Studies on Cardiac Structure and Metabolism*, edited by A. Fleckenstein and G. Rona. Baltimore, MD: University Park, 1975, vol. 6, p. 325–333.
8. HORIBA, N., K. NOMURA, Y. SAITO, H. DEMURA, AND K. SHIZUME. Rat atrial natriuretic polypeptide stimulation of adrenal zona glomerulosa cell growth. *Biochem. Biophys. Res. Commun.* 132: 261–263, 1985.
9. KELLY, F. J., AND D. F. GOLDSPINK. The differing responses of four muscle types to dexamethasone treatment in the rat. *Biochem. J.* 208: 147–151, 1982.
10. LANG, R. E., H. THÖLKEN, D. GANTEN, F. C. LUFT, H. RUSKOAHO, AND T. UNGER. Atrial natriuretic factor—a circulating hormone stimulated by volume loading. *Nature Lond.* 314: 264–266, 1985.
11. LEAK, L. V., AND J. F. BURKE. The ultrastructure of human embryonic myocardium. *Anat. Rec.* 149: 623–650, 1964.
12. MANNING, P. T., D. SCHWARTZ, N. C. KATSUBE, S. W. HOLMBERG, AND P. NEEDLEMAN. Vasopressin-stimulated release of atriopeptin: endocrine antagonists in fluid homeostasis. *Science Wash. DC* 229: 395–397, 1985.
13. MATSUO, H., K. KANGAWA, AND A. MIYATA. Atrial natriuretic polypeptides (ANP): molecular forms and distribution in mammalian tissues and plasma. In: *Peptides: Structure and*

Function, edited by C. M. Deber, V. J. Hruby, and K. D. Kopple. Rockford, IL: Pierce Chem., 1985, p. 925–932.

14. MORII, N., K. NAKAO, A. SUGAWARA, M. SAKAMOTO, M. SUDA, M. SHIMOKURA, Y. KISO, M. KIHARA, Y. YAMORI, AND H. IMURA. Occurrence of atrial natriuretic polypeptide in brain. *Biochem. Biophys. Res. Commun.* 127: 413–419, 1985.

15. NAKAYAMA, K., H. OHKUBO, T. HIROSE, S. INAYAMA, AND S. NAKANISHI. mRNA sequence for human cardiodilatin-atrial natriuretic factor precursor and regulation of precursor mRNA in rat atria. *Nature Lond.* 310: 699–701, 1984.

16. NAPIER, M. A., R. L. VANDLEN, G. ALBERS-SCHÖNBERG, R. F. NUTT, S. BRADY, T. LYLE, R. WINQUEST, E. P. FAISON, L. A. HEINEL, AND E. H. BLAINE. Specific membrane receptors for atrial natriuretic factor in renal and vascular tissues. *Proc. Natl. Acad. Sci. USA* 81: 5946–5950, 1984.

17. NEEDLEMAN, P., S. P. ADAMS, B. R. COLE, M. G. CURRIE, D. M. GELLER, M. L. MICHENER, C. B. SAPER, D. SCHWARTZ, AND D. G. STANDAERT. Atriopeptins as cardiac hormones. *Hypertension Dallas* 7: 469–482, 1985.

18. SAKAMOTO, M., K. NAKAO, M. KIHARA, N. MORII, A. SUGAWARA, M. SUDA, M. SHIMOKURA, Y. KISO, Y. YAMORI, AND H. IMURA. Existence of atrial natriuretic polypeptide in kidney. *Biochem. Biophys. Res. Commun.* 128: 1281–1287, 1985.

19. SCHWARTZ, D., D. M. GELLER, P. T. MANNING, N. R. SIEGEL, K. F. FOK, C. E. SMITH, AND P. NEEDLEMAN. Ser-Leu-Arg-Arg-atriopeptin III: the major circulating form of atrial peptide. *Science Wash DC* 229: 397–400, 1985.

20. SEIDMAN, C. E., K. D. BLOCH, K. A. KLEIN, J. A. SMITH, AND J. G. SEIDMAN. Nucleotide sequences of the human and mouse atrial natriuretic factor genes. *Science Wash. DC* 226: 1206–1209, 1984.

21. SELEZNEV, I. M., A. A. SHNYRA, S. M. DANILOV, AND G. V. KOLPAKOVA. Heterogeneity of cardiac glucocorticoid receptors. *Biull. Vsesoiuznogo Kardiol. Nauchn. Tsentra* 4: 18–22, 1981.

22. STONE, R. A., AND C. G. GLEMBOTSKI. Immunoreactive atrial natriuretic peptide in the rat eye: molecular forms in the anterior uvea and retina. *Biochem. Biophys. Res. Commun.* 134: 1022–1028, 1986.

23. TAKAYANAGI, R., I. TANAKA, M. MAKI, AND T. INAGAMI. Effects of changes in water-sodium balance on levels of atrial natriuretic factor messenger RNA and peptide in rats. *Life Sci.* 36: 1843–1848, 1985.

24. THIBAULT, G., C. LAZURE, E. L. SCHIFFRIN, J. GUTKOWSKA, L. CHARTIER, R. GARCIA, N. G. SEIDAH, M. CHRÉTIEN, J. GENEST, AND M. CANTIN. Identification of a biologically active circulating form of rat atrial natriuretic factor. *Biochem. Biophys. Res. Commun.* 130: 981–986, 1985.

25. ZIVIN, R. A., J. H. CONDRA, R. A. F. DIXON, N. G. SEIDAH, M. CHRÉTIEN, M. NEMER, M. CHAMBERLAND, AND J. DROUIN. Molecular cloning and characterization of DNA sequences encoding rat and human atrial naturiuretic factors. *Proc. Natl. Acad. Sci. USA* 81: 6325–6329, 1984.

5

Tissue Distribution of Atrial Natriuretic Factor and Determination of Its Concentration

TADASHI INAGAMI, TERUAKI IMADA, ISSEI TANAKA,
RYOICHI TAKAYANAGI, MITSUHIDE NARUSE,
RICHARD J. RODEHEFFER, ALAN S. HOLLISTER,
AND KUNIO S. MISONO

*Departments of Biochemistry and Medicine, Vanderbilt University School
of Medicine, Nashville, Tennessee; and Department of Internal
Medicine, Tokyo Women's Medical College, Tokyo, Japan*

Radioimmunoassay of Atrial Natriuretic Factor (ANF)
Elevation of Plasma ANF Levels Under Various Pathophysiological Conditions
Atrial Natriuretic Factor in Extra-Atrial Organs
Molecular Properties of ANF

TO DETERMINE THE LOCALIZATION and concentration of atrial natriuretic factor (ANF) in various tissues, we produced antibodies to ANF and determined ANF by the immunohistochemical method and radioimmunoassay. The assay of ANF in plasma required extraction of the peptide either by solid-phase adsorbents or solvents. Plasma ANF values determined in various laboratories vary widely but are beginning to converge to consensus values. Plasma ANF has been found markedly elevated in various hypertensive rats, in the plasma of subjects with essential hypertension, and in advanced states of congestive heart failure. These results coupled with good correlation between cardiac and pulmonary blood pressure and plasma ANF concentration indicate that atrial blood pressure, hence atrial distension, may be the major controlling factor in the stimulation of ANF secretion. In addition to atria, ANF was found in the ventricle, brain, anterior pituitary, thyroid gland, submandibular gland, adrenal medulla, and peripheral nerves. Local functions of these peripherally localized ANF are envisaged. The ANF in circulation was identified as a low-molecular-weight form with 28 amino acid residues, whereas ANF stored in the atrium is mostly proANF with 126 amino acid residues. Conversion seems to take place at the time of secretion. On the other hand, ANF in other tissues such as the ventricle and hypothalamus is the low-molecular-weight form. The mechanism involved in the conversion of proANF to the low-molecular-weight form is not known.

RADIOIMMUNOASSAY OF ANF

Atrial natriuretic factor was recognized by its natriuretic, diuretic, and vasorelaxant activity in the extract of the atrium. The evaluation of its

39

pathophysiological roles required the determination of its concentration in plasma and tissues under various pathophysiological conditions. While bioassay methods were used in the early stage of ANF research, these methods were quickly replaced by the radioimmunoassay method because of rapid progress in the purification of ANF and determination of its structure.

Based on the structural information of rat (37, 38) and human (25) ANF, we have synthesized 25–amino acid ANF peptides of the rat and human (65) and used them to produce specific antibodies to ANF in rabbits. Application of the antibodies to radioimmunoassay of ANF was developed in 1984 (69). The assay depends on synthetic ANF radioiodinated at the COOH-terminal tyrosine residue. Since this work and that of Gutkowska et al. (16), similar methods have been developed in many laboratories (2, 8, 14, 18, 28, 29, 39, 45, 53, 74, 77). Although some methods were for tissue extracts, many of these techniques were applicable to the determination of plasma ANF. Earlier, delayed addition of radioactive tracer was used to enhance the sensitivity of the assay. This method, compared with simultaneous addition of the tracer and sample, improves the sensitivity of assay by a factor of 2–3. As the quality of antibodies has been improved, the use of simultaneous addition has become more prevalent. The separation of antibody-bound tracer and free tracer can be accomplished by charcoal treatment, by polyethylene glycol in the presence of rabbit immunoglobulin G (IgG), or by secondary antibodies. The latter two methods seem to give a more satisfactory separation than charcoal.

Although tissue extract can be subjected to the radioimmunoassay without additional treatment or "extraction," plasma samples require the extraction. Without the extraction, artificially higher values were obtained (77), often 5–10 times greater than the value obtained with extracted plasma samples. This is illustrated in Figure 1 with results obtained by K. Abe (unpublished observations). Solid-phase extraction can be performed with a Sep-Pak C_{18}

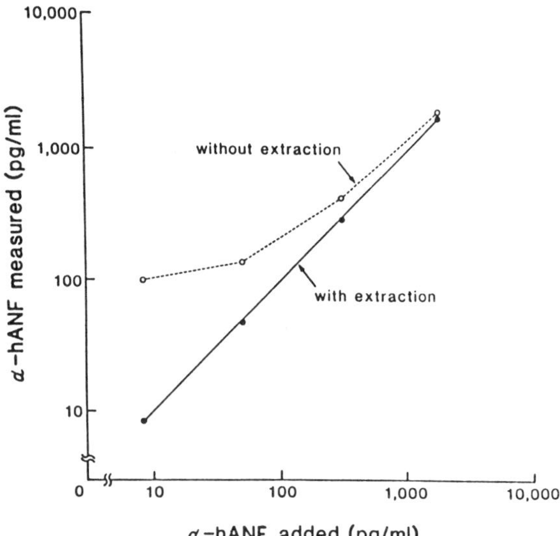

FIG. 1. Comparison of results of radioimmunoassay of human atrial natriuretic factor (hANF) with or without extraction by a column containing immunoaffinity Sepharose. Synthetic hANF was mixed with human plasma freed from ANF by passage through the immunoaffinity gel and used as samples. (Courtesy of K. Abe.)

cartridge (20, 28, 29, 39, 45, 69), Vycor glass beads (14), immunoaffinity gel (14, 74, 77), or Amberlite XAD-2 resin (2). Extraction with solvents such as methanol and chloroform is equally effective in removing interfering substances in plasma.

The solid-phase extraction method has been simplified. The method currently used in our laboratory is briefly described here. A Sep-Pak C_{18} cartridge is washed with methanol (20 ml) and 0.1 M acetic acid (20 ml). Plasma (2 ml) mixed with 1 ml of 0.3 M acetic acid is applied to it, and the cartridge is washed with 20 ml of 0.1 M acetic acid. The ANF is eluted with 3 ml of 80% methanol. After evaporating methanol in a vacuum centrifuge followed by lyophilization, residues are dissolved in 1 ml of radioimmunoassay buffer.

The solvent extraction is performed by mixing 1 ml of plasma with 3.0 ml of methanol and 1.5 ml of chloroform. The mixture is stirred well by vortexing. After standing for 30 min at 4°C, it is centrifuged for 15 min at 2,000 g and the supernatant is separated from protein precipitates. Chloroform (3 ml) and water (1.5 ml) are added to the supernatant, mixed well, and allowed to stand for 30 min at 4°C. After centrifugation for 15 min at 2,000 g the upper layer is collected by pipetting. The solvent is evaporated in a vacuum centrifuge, and the remaining aqueous phase is lyophilized. The dried residue is dissolved in radioimmunoassay buffer that consists of 0.1 M Tris-acetate, pH 7.4, 0.1% bovine serum albumin, 1 mM ethylenediaminetetraacetate (EDTA), 0.02% sodium azide, 500 U/ml aprotinin, and 500 U/ml soybean trypsin inhibitor.

In the radioimmunoassay, sample or standard (0.1 ml) is incubated with appropriately diluted antiserum (0.1 ml), ^{125}I-labeled ANF (0.1 ml), and 0.3 ml of the assay buffer for 24 h at 4°C. Free and antibody-bound radiotracer were separated by adding 0.18 ml of 1% bovine γ-globulin and 0.7 ml of 25% polyethylene glycol [molecular weight (MW) 8,000] followed by centrifugation for 30 min at 3,000 g. Supernatant was aspirated off and radioactivity in the sediment was counted. With this method and the use of specific anti-human ANF or anti-rat ANF antisera, 0.5–3 pg of ANF can be detected.

By the application of the radioimmunoassay to rat plasma we were able to demonstrate ANF in blood (69). This observation was the first indication that ANF is a circulating hormone, a conclusion supported by many subsequent studies. As is usually the case with the development of radioimmunoassay methods, the plasma ANF values determined earlier were high, and as the assay was improved, normal plasma values were gradually reduced. By the current consensus the average plasma ANF in normal rat is 50–150 pg/ml of plasma (Table 1). The plasma value is influenced profoundly by ether anesthesia, whereas pentobarbital tends to somewhat reduce the plasma ANF levels (19) or affects it very little in our experience.

ELEVATION OF PLASMA ANF LEVELS UNDER VARIOUS PATHOPHYSIOLOGICAL CONDITIONS

Elevation of blood pressure in certain hypertensive rats was found to be accompanied by increased plasma ANF levels (Table 2). We found that plasma

TABLE 1. *Levels of ANF in rat plasma*

ANF, pg/ml	Rat	Anesthesia	Extraction	Ref.
1,250 ± 210	Sprague-Dawley	Ether	Antibody-Sepharose	14
1,020 ± 110	Sprague-Dawley	Ether	Vycor glass	14
421 ± 37	Sprague-Dawley	Pentobarbital	Sep-Pak C_{18}	69
389 ± 53	Wistar		Sep-Pak C_{18}	39
172 ± 19	Wistar-Kyoto	Pentobarbital	Sep-Pak C_{18}	20
170 ± 17	Wistar-Kyoto	Pentobarbital	Sep-Pak C_{18}	41
125 ± 16	Sprague-Dawley		Sep-Pak C_{18}	8
120 ± 8	Dahl salt-resistant	Pentobarbital	Sep-Pak C_{18}	67
101 ± 10	Sprague-Dawley	Conscious	Sep-Pak C_{18}	35
94 ± 17	Sprague-Dawley	Conscious	Vycor glass	19
55 ± 14	Wistar		Octadecylsilane	28

ANF, atrial natriuretic factor.

TABLE 2. *Atrial natriuretic factor in plasma of hypertensive rats*

Hypertensive	ANF, pg/ml	Normotensive	ANF, pg/ml	Ref.
Spontaneously hypertensive, 16 wk	451 ± 48	Wistar-Kyoto	172 ± 19	20
Dahl salt-sensitive	238 ± 46	Dahl salt-resistant	109 ± 7.8	67
Pulmonary hypertension	238 ± 107	Control	101 ± 10	35

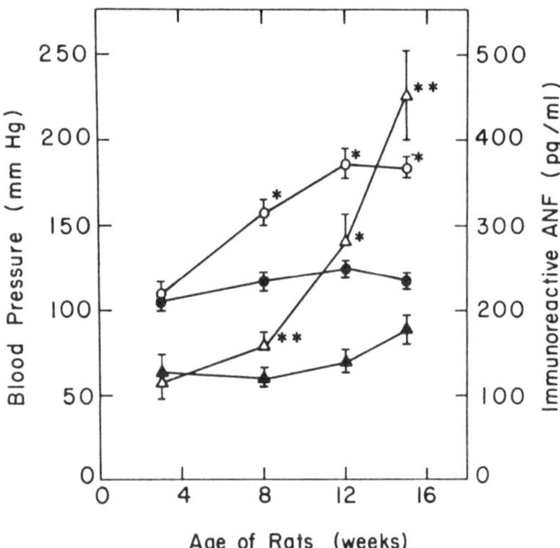

FIG. 2. Plasma levels of immuno-reactive atrial natriuretic factor (ANF) in plasma of spontaneously hypertensive rats (SHR, △) and Wistar-Kyoto (WKY, ▲) rats. Blood pressure of SHR (○) and WKY (●) was also measured. * $P < 0.01$; ** $P < 0.05$. [From Imada et al. (20).]

ANF of spontaneously hypertensive rats (SHR) was increased with age and blood pressure (Fig. 2; 20). The elevated plasma ANF levels in SHR and their stroke-prone substrain were also reported by Morii et al. (41). The plasma ANF level of Dahl salt-sensitive (S) rats was markedly elevated with the development of hypertension on a high-salt diet (67). Likewise, pulmonary hypertension caused a more than twofold elevation in plasma ANF (35). In view of reports from several laboratories that the secretion of ANF is stimu-

TABLE 3. *Concentration of ANF in various rat organs*

			Ref.
Atrium, right*	1,550	± 320	20
	468	± 63	40
Atrium, left*	1,210	± 100	20
	263	± 19	40
Ventricle†	0.012	± 0.002	66
	0.31	± 0.11	40
Submandibular gland†	0.241	± 0.039	40
Thyroid gland†	0.095	± 0.0096	40
Brain, hypothalamus†	0.015	± 0.002	69
Brain, whole†	0.0060	± 0.0005	40
Adrenal gland†	0.07	± 0.004‡	
	0.0056	± 0.0006	40
Plasma§	101	± 10	35
	389	± 53	40

*Equivalent of proANF, ng/mg wet tissue.　　†Equivalent of 28 residue ANF, ng/mg wet tissue.　　‡Unpublished observations of I. Tanaka.　　§28 Residue ANF, pg/ml.

TABLE 4. *Levels of ANF in human plasma*

ANF, pg/ml	Extraction	Ref.
231 ± 37	Sep-Pak C_{18}	39
127 ± 77	Sep-Pak C_{18}	48
86.7 ± 9.3	Sep-Pak C_{18}	51
65.3 ± 2.5	Vycor glass	13
59.1 ± 9.3		76
44.6 ± 3.7	C_{18} cartridge	4
37.7 ± 7.0	Sep-Pak C_{18}	64
37.6 ± 24.4	ANF antibody-Sepharose	46
26.7 ± 7.2	Amberlite XAD-2	2
22.4 ± 6.2	Sep-Pak C_{18}	29
20.0 ± 4.0	Sep-Pak C_{18}	17
10.0 ± 3.1	Direct	72
8.4 ± 3.7	Sep-Pak C_{18}	54

lated by atrial distension, the elevation of plasma seems to be a result of hypertension rather than the cause of hypertension (7, 28, 31). Atrial tissue levels of ANF were not as markedly affected by hypertension. As atrial tissue levels of ANF were increased with age, those of SHR in the left atrium were lower than those of the control Wistar-Kyoto (WKY) strain. The left atrium of the rat contains less ANF than the right atrium (Table 3; 20).

The basal ANF levels of peripheral plasma in human subjects reported by several investigators are summarized in Table 4. Although the ANF content in human plasma was much more variable than in rats, the human plasma concentration was lower than that of the rat. It seems to be affected strongly by salt intake, blood pressure, and posture. Hollister et al. (17) found that plasma ANF increment due to salt intake is strongly correlated with body weight increase, which may be directly related to fluid volume expansion. Relationship with salt intake was also reported by several investigators (18, 53, 72). Direct relationship of plasma ANF levels to the blood pressure in the central circulation in patients with a variety of heart diseases was investigated by Rodeheffer et al. (52). Good correlations were found between right atrial pressure and pulmonary artery ANF concentration as well as between pulmonary capillary wedge pressure and aorta ANF concentration (52). Furthermore, acute alteration in atrial pressure correlated directly with prompt changes in ANF concentration (52). Several investigators found that the plasma of patients with congestive heart failure, particularly those in stages III and IV (defined by the New York Heart Association), contained markedly elevated ANF concentrations (Fig. 3; 4, 46, 52). These observations coupled with the elevated ANF levels in hypertensive rats (20, 35, 41, 67) support the view that ANF is released in response to the elevated fluid volume or blood pressure to alleviate the work load of the heart.

In human essential hypertension, plasma ANF is elevated (54). However, in many subjects the plasma ANF level was within a normal range (48) and not a diagnostically useful index for essential hypertension. Plasma ANF is markedly elevated in cirrhosis (48). On the other hand, in idiopathic edematous

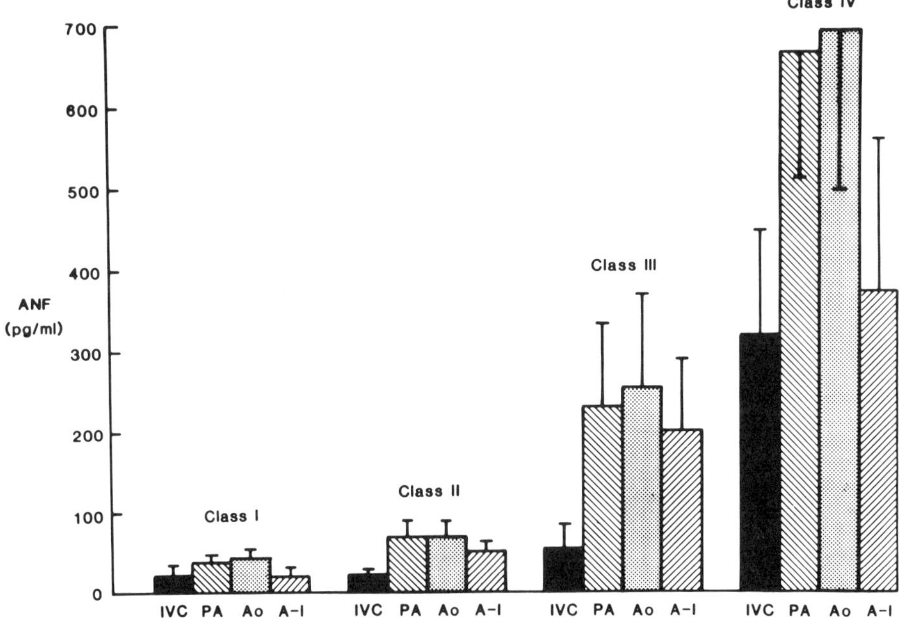

FIG. 3. Plasma levels of immunoreactive atrial natriuretic factor (ANF) in plasma of patients with various degrees of congestive heart failure classified according to New York Heart Association. Levels of ANF were measured in plasma obtained from the inferior vena cava (IVC), pulmonary artery (PA), and aorta (Ao). Difference between ANF levels in the aorta and inferior vena cava (A − I) were estimated as a measure for rate of secretion of ANF from the heart. [Data from Rodeheffer et al. (52).]

patients, ANF is not significantly elevated, despite volume loading (48). The edema may be due to a defective mechanism of ANF secretion in response to volume expansion.

Although both right and left atria contain ANF, its content per wet weight tissue is greater in the right atrium of rat than in the left atrium (Table 3). Among the various tissues the content of ANF is the highest in the atria, and both left and right atria seem to be the major source of circulating ANF. However, the presence of ANF is not limited to the atria. We have observed that the ventricle also contains a small amount of ANF, 1/10,000 of the amount in the atria (Table 3). Because the ventricle also contains mRNA for ANF, which can be hybridized with ANF cDNA (66), it is highly likely that ANF in the ventricle is synthesized locally rather than being taken up from the plasma and accumulated in the ventricle.

ATRIAL NATRIURETIC FACTOR IN EXTRA-ATRIAL ORGANS

The presence of ANF is not limited to the heart (Table 3). Application of the radioimmunoassay led us to the discovery of ANF in the brain of the rat (69). In the brain, ANF was most concentrated in the hypothalamus. Morii et al. (42) surveyed various areas of rat brain by microdissection using a radioimmunoassay and reported that the hypothalamus and septum are the highest in ANF concentration, followed by midbrain, cortex, olfactory bulb, thalamus, and the pontine-medullary region. Zamir et al. (78) used punches from frozen sections to determine ANF content in various regions of rat brain. Extensive regions were studied. Atrial natriuretic factor was found in a variety of regions in circumventricular organs; telencephalic, diencephalic, mesencephalic regions; medulla oblongata; and spinal cord. These regions included the thalamus, hypothalamus, hippocampus, amygdala, dorsal raphe nucleus, locus coeruleus periaqueductal gray, organum vasculosum of the lamina terminalis, subfornical organ, and area postrema.

The concentration of ANF in the brain is very low. The highest concentration (10–20 ng/g wet tissue) was found in the hypothalamus (20, 42, 69, 78). However, it is 10,000 times less than that in the atria. The ANF is distributed over a wide range of the brain tissue. Immunohistochemical staining of ANF in the brain supports these observations. The ANF-containing neurons were localized in preoptic and hypothalamic neurons (21, 57) and neurons in the mesencephalon and pons (57). Detailed studies combining immunohistochemical localization and microdissection radioimmunoassay have been reported by Kawata et al. (27). Neurons that were prominently stained by antibodies to ANF were the ventral region of lateral septal nucleus, periventricular preoptic nucleus, red nucleus of the stria terminalis, periventricular and dorsal regions of the paraventricular nucleus, ventromedial nucleus, dorsomedial nucleus, arcuate nucleus, median mamillary nucleus, supramamillary nucleus, zona incerta, medial habenular nucleus, and the periaqueductal gray matter. Scattered immunopositive nuclei were in the cingulate cortex, endopiriform nucleus, lateral hypothalamic area, and pretectal and dorsal thalamic areas. Immunoreactive varicose fibers were seen in the glomerular layer of the olfactory bulb, external layer of the median eminence, central to paramedian regions of interpeduncular nucleus, and the paraventricular hypothalamic nucleus. Considerable numbers of immunoreactive varicose fibers were also observed in globus pallidus, medial and central amygdaloid nuclei, dorsal raphe nucleus, dorsal parabrachial nucleus, locus coeruleus, vagal dorsal motor nucleus, solitary nucleus, subfornical organ, and organum vasculosum laminae terminalis.

The presence of ANF in perikarya of the neuronal cells suggests its local synthesis. Indeed our preliminary studies indicate the presence of mRNA for ANF in the brain. The ANF in the brain has been shown to be secretable in in vitro experiments that use potassium-induced depolarization (60, 68).

The finding that ANF is localized in various brain regions, including various nuclei inside the blood-brain barrier, indicates that brain ANF may function in the brain independent of the circulating ANF. The ANF administered into cerebral ventricles was found to inhibit angiotensin II–induced or dehydration-induced dipsogenesis in rats (1, 33, 43, 44).

Atrial natriuretic factor has been found to inhibit vasopressin release in dehydrated or hemorrhaging rats (55) or vasopressin release from neurohypophysis in vitro (23, 49); ANF was also reported to stimulate vasopressin release (22). Immunohistochemical studies also revealed the presence of ANF in the anterior pituitary (36). In in vitro studies ANF was found to suppress the secretion of ACTH, β-endorphin, and γ-MSH (melanocyte-stimulating hormone) as well as growth hormone. Thus ANF may have some local action in the central nervous system and the pituitary.

In addition to its presence in the brain, ANF has been reported in peripheral nerve. By radioimmunoassay, immunoreactive ANF was found in parasympathetic ganglia of rats (6).

The levels of ANF in the brain are reduced by salt feeding, contrary to plasma or atrial ANF levels, which are increased by salt feeding (69), again indicating the independence of brain ANF from circulating ANF. The ANF in several hypothalmic regions in the rat is markedly reduced by dehydration (56).

In addition to the atria, ventricle, and brain, immunoreactive ANF has been reported in the retina (63), chorion (A. Poisner and T. Imada, unpublished observations), and testis. Immunohistochemical studies also revealed its presence in adrenomedullary chromaffin cells, anterior pituitary cells, and intercalated cells of the renal collecting duct of rats (35).

MOLECULAR PROPERTIES OF ANF

Although ANFs of various chain lengths have been isolated from the atria of the heart, later studies conducted with specific care to minimize the degradation of ANF during extraction indicate that immunoreactive ANF in rat atrium is predominantly in high-molecular-weight form (12, 20, 39, 64, 69,

73). Various investigators have isolated the high-molecular-weight ANFs and determined their structures. Peptides with 73 (70), 106 (30), 111 (10), and 126 (26) amino acid residues or their fragments were purified and their amino acid sequences were determined. In view of the greatest abundance of the peptide with 126 amino acid residues in rat atrium (26), it is now considered as the major storage form of rat atrium. The smaller precursors seem to be the artifact of proteolytic degradation. The agreement of its amino acid sequence determined directly with purified γ-rat ANP (γ-atrial natriuretic polypeptide) agreed with that of proANF inferred from the amino acid sequence of preproANF that was deduced from the base sequence of the cDNA of ANF (32, 47, 59, 75). The synthesis and presence of this 126–amino acid residue peptide were also demonstrated in the primary culture of rat atriocyte (3, 11). Thus it is now agreed that proANF is the storage form of ANF in the rat atrium. The proANF (γ-ANP) from human atrium was also isolated in a pure form, and its amino acid sequence was determined by Kangawa et al. (24). Again its structure was in agreement with that of the proANF portion deduced from the base sequence of its cDNA (50). Human atrium seems to contain proANF as well as low-molecular-weight ANF (α-ANP and β-ANP, a dimer of α-ANP) (24, 50).

The circulating form of ANF in plasma has been shown to be a low-molecular-weight form (12, 20, 39, 64, 69, 73). Krebs-Ringer perfused heart also releases the low-molecular-weight form (5). Schwartz et al. (58) and Thibault et al. (71) have purified the circulating form from rat plasma with immunoaffinity chromatography and determined its amino acid sequence. It was identified as the 28–amino acid residue peptide identical with cardionatrin purified and sequenced by Flynn et al. (9) with the structure

Ser-Leu-Arg-Arg-Ser-Ser-Cys-Phe-Gly-Gly-Arg-Ile-Asp-Arg-Ile-Gly-
|
Ala-Gln-Ser-Gly-Leu-Gly-Cys-Asn-Ser-Phe-Arg-Tyr

A low-molecular-weight peptide was also recognized in human plasma as the circulating form (29, 64).

These findings indicated that ANF is synthesized as preproANF with 152 amino acid residues, processed to proANF with 126 amino acid residues, and stored in this prohormone form. However, when it is secreted it is converted to the low-molecular-weight form with 28–amino acid residue peptide. The mechanism of this conversion is not clear. The proANF formed and stored in cultured rat atriocytes was found to be secreted intact without being processed (3, 11). These findings do not agree with the observations of the low-molecular-weight ANF in plasma or the Krebs-Ringer perfusate of the heart. On the other hand, Gutkowska et al. (15) have reported that ANF (Arg101-Tyr126) is secreted from cultured rat atriocytes. At this point this discrepancy cannot be explained.

We found that ANF in the ventricle of the heart is a mixture of proANF and the low-molecular-weight form; the latter is predominant (66). On the other hand, Miyata et al. (40) reported that ventricular ANF is the large form (proANF). We have shown that ANF in the brain consists of a small form and an intermediate form, as assessed by gel filtration (69). A later study using reverse-phase HPLC (high-performance liquid chromatography) and gel-permeation HPLC showed that brain ANF consists entirely of several small forms containing 28 or fewer amino acid residues (20). Similar observations were reported by Morii et al. (42) and Glembotski et al. (12). Shiono et al. (62) have reported that brain ANF consists of 25 and 24 residue peptides. Thus, in the brain, ANF seems to be processed and stored in neurons before secretion. Our in vitro studies on the secretion of ANF from rat hypothalamus showed that a peptide containing less than 28 amino acid residues but more than 25 residues is secreted to a depolarizing medium (68). Peptidases different from that in the atrium seem to be responsible for the conversion of proANF to the smaller forms. The mechanism of the conversion also seems to be different.

We thank Dr. K. Abe of the National Cancer Center of Japan for his unpublished results and Steve Richardson for typing the manuscript.

This work was supported by grants from the National Institutes of Health (HL-35323, HL-14192, HL-31419, and RR-00095) and the American Heart Association (84-1291).

REFERENCES

1. ANTUNES-RODRIGUES, J., S. M. MCCANN, L. C. ROGERS, AND W. K. SAMSON. Atrial natriuretic factor inhibits dehydration- and angiotensin II-induced water intake in the conscious, unrestrained rat. *Proc. Natl. Acad. Sci. USA* 82: 8720–8723, 1985.

2. ARENDT, R. M., E. STANGEL, J. ZÄHRINGER, D. C. LIEBISCH, AND A. HERZ. Demonstration and characterization of α-human atrial natriuretic factor in human plasma. *FEBS Lett.* 189: 57–61, 1985.

3. BLOCH, K. D., J. A. SCOTT, J. B. ZISTEIN, J. T. FALLON, M. N. MARGOLIES, C. E. SEIDMAN, G. R. MATSUEDA, C. HOMCY, R. M. GRAHAM, AND J. G. SEIDMAN. Biosynthesis and secretion of proatrial natriuretic factor by cultured rat cardiocytes. *Science Wash. DC* 230: 1168–1171, 1985.

4. BURNETT, J. C., P. C. KAO, D. C. HU, D. W. HESER, D. HEUBLEIN, J. P. GRANGER, T. J. OPGENROTH, AND G. S. REEDER. Atrial natriuretic peptide elevation in congestive heart failure in the human. *Science Wash. DC* 231: 1145–1147, 1986.

5. CURRIE, M. G., D. SUKIN, D. M. GELLER, B. R. COLE, AND P. NEEDLEMAN. Atriopeptin release from the isolated perfused rabbit heart. *Biochem. Biophys. Res. Commun.* 124: 711–717, 1984.

6. DEBINSKY, W., J. GUTKOWSKA, O. KUCHEL, K. RACZ, N. T. BUU, M. CANTIN, AND J. GENEST. ANF-like peptide(s) in the peripheral autonomic nervous system. *Biochem. Biophys. Res. Commun.* 134: 279–284, 1986.

7. DIETZ, J. R. Release of natriuretic factor from rat heart-lung preparation by atrial distension. *Am. J. Physiol.* 247 (*Regulatory Integrative Comp. Physiol.* 16): R1093–R1096, 1984.

8. ESKAY, R., Z. ZUKOWSKA-GROJEC, M. HAASS, J. R. DAVE, AND N. ZAMIR. Circulating atrial natriuretic peptides in conscious rats: regulation of release by multiple factors. *Science Wash. DC* 232: 636–639, 1986.

9. FLYNN, T. G., M. L. DE BOLD, AND A. J. DE BOLD. The amino acid sequence of an atrial peptide with potent diuretic and natriuretic properties. *Biochem. Biophys. Res. Commun.* 117: 859–865, 1983.

10. GELLER, D. M., M. G. CURRIE, N. R. SIEGEL, K. F. FOK, S. P. ADAMS, AND P. NEEDLEMAN. The sequence of atriopeptigen: a precursor of the bioactive atrial peptides. *Biochem. Biophys. Res. Commun.* 121: 802–807, 1984.

11. GLEMBOTSKI, C. C., AND T. R. GIBSON. Molecular forms of immunoreactive atrial natriuretic peptide released from cultured rat atrial myocytes. *Biochem. Biophys. Res. Commun.* 132: 1008–1017, 1985.

12. GLEMBOTSKI, C. C., G. M. WILDEY, AND T. R. GIBSON. Molecular forms of immunoactive

atrial natriuretic peptide in the rat hypothalamus and atrium. *Biochem. Biophys. Res. Commun.* 129: 671–678, 1985.

13. GUTKOWSKA, J., M. BOURASSA, D. ROY, G. THIBAULT, R. GARCIA, M. CANTIN, AND J. GENEST. Immunoreactive atrial natriuretic factor (IR-ANF) in human plasma. *Biochem. Biophys. Res. Commun.* 128: 1350–1357, 1985.

14. GUTKOWSKA, J., K. HORKÝ, G. THIBAULT, P. JANUSZEWICA, M. CANTIN, AND J. GENEST. Atrial natriuretic factor is a circulating hormone. *Biochem. Biophys. Res. Commun.* 125: 315–323, 1984.

15. GUTKOWSKA, J., C. LAZURE, K. RACZ, G. THIBAULT, R. GARCIA, N. G. SEIDAH, M. CHRÉTIEN, J. GENEST, AND M. CANTIN. ANF (Arg 101-Tyr 126) is the peptide secreted by rat atrial cardiocytes in culture. *Biochem. Biophys. Res. Commun.* 130: 1217–1225, 1985.

16. GUTKOWSKA, J., G. THIBAULT, R. W. MILNE, P. JANUSZEWICZ, P. W. SCHILLER, M. CANTIN, AND J. GENEST. Radioimmunoassay of atrial natriuretic factor (ANF) in rat atria. *Proc. Soc. Exp. Biol. Med.* 176: 105–108, 1984.

17. HOLLISTER, A. S., I. TANAKA, T. IMADA, J. ONROT, I. BIAGIONI, D. ROBERTSON, AND T. INAGAMI. Modulation of plasma atrial natriuretic factor levels in human subjects by sodium loading and posture change. *Hypertension Dallas* 8, Suppl. II: II102–II111, 1986.

18. HOMCY, C., R. GAIVIN, J. ZISFEIN, AND R. M. GRAHAM. Snack-induced release of atrial natriuretic factor. *N. Engl. J. Med.* 313: 1484, 1985.

19. HORKY, K., J. GUTKOWSKA, R. GARCIA, G. THIBAULT, J. GENEST, AND M. CANTIN. Effect of different anesthetics on immunoreactive atrial natriuretic factor concentrations in rat plasma. *Biochem. Biophys. Res. Commun.* 129: 651–657, 1985.

20. IMADA, T., R. TAKAYANAGI, AND T. INAGAMI. Changes in the content of atrial natriuretic factor with the progression of hypertension in spontaneously hypertensive rats. *Biochem. Biophys. Res. Commun.* 133: 759–765, 1985.

21. JACOBOWITZ, D. M., G. SKOFITSCH, H. R. KEISER, R. L. ESKAY, AND N. ZAMIR. Evidence for the existence of atrial natriuretic factor-containing neurons in the rat brain. *Neuroendocrinology* 40: 92–94, 1985.

22. JANUSZEWICZ, P., J. GUTKOWSKA, A. DE LÉAN, G. THIBAULT, R. GARCIA, J. GENEST, AND M. CANTIN. Synthetic atrial natriuretic factor induces release (possibly receptor-mediated) of vasopressin from rat posterior pituitary. *Proc. Soc. Exp. Biol. Med.* 178: 321–325, 1985.

23. JANUSZEWICZ, P., G. THIBAULT, R. GARCIA, J. GUTKOWSKA, J. GENEST, AND M. CANTIN. Effect of synthetic atrial natriuretic factor on arginine vasopressin release by the rat hypothalamoneurohypophysial complex in organ culture. *Biochem. Biophys. Res. Commun.* 134: 652–658, 1986.

24. KANGAWA, K., A. FUKUDA, AND H. MATSUO. Structural identification of β- and γ-human atrial natriuretic polypeptides. *Nature Lond.* 313: 397–400, 1985.

25. KANGAWA, K., AND H. MATSUO. Purification and complete amino acid sequence of alpha human atrial natriuretic polypeptide (alpha-hANP). *Biochem. Biophys. Res. Commun.* 118: 131–139, 1984.

26. KANGAWA, K., Y. TAWARAGI, S. OIKAWA, A. MIZUNO, Y. SAKURAGAWA, H. NAKAZATO, A. FUKUDA, N. MINAMINO, AND H. MATSUO. Identification of rat gamma atrial natriuretic polypeptide and characterization of the cDNA encoding its precursor. *Nature Lond.* 312: 152–155, 1984.

27. KAWATA, M., K. NAKAO, N. MORII, Y. KISO, H. YAMASHITA, H. IMURA, AND Y. SANO. Atrial natriuretic polypeptide: topographical distribution in the rat brain by radioimmunoassay and immunohistochemistry. *Neuroscience* 16: 521–546, 1985.

28. LANG, R. E., H. THÖLKEN, D. GANTEN, F. C. LUFT, H. RUSKOAHO, AND T. UNGAR. Atrial natriuretic factor—a circulating hormone stimulated by volume loading. *Nature Lond.* 314: 264–266, 1985.

29. LAROSE, P., S. MELOCHE, P. DU SOUICH, A. DE LÉAN, AND H. ONG. Radioimmunoassay of atrial natriuretic factor: human plasma levels. *Biochem. Biophys. Res. Commun.* 130: 553–558, 1985.

30. LAZURE, C., N. G. SEIDAH, M. CHRÉTIEN, G. THIBAULT, R. GARCIA, M. CANTIN, AND J. GENEST. Atrial pronatriodilatin: a precursor for natriuretic factor and cardiodilatin. Amino acid sequence evidence. *FEBS Lett.* 172: 80–86, 1984.

31. LEDSOME, J. R., N. WILSON, C. A. COURNEYA, AND A. J. RANKIN. Release of atrial natriuretic peptide by atrial distension. *Can. J. Physiol. Pharmacol.* 63: 739–742, 1985.

32. MAKI, M., R. TAKAYANAGI, K. S. MISONO, K. N. PANDEY, C. TIBBETTS, AND T. INAGAMI.

Structure of rat atrial natriuretic factor precursor deduced from cDNA sequence. *Nature Lond.* 309: 722–724, 1984.

33. MASOTTO, C., AND A. NEGRO-VILAR. Inhibition of spontaneous or angiotensin II-stimulated water intake by atrial natriuretic factor. *Brain Res. Bull.* 15: 523–526, 1985.

34. MATSUO, H., AND K. KANAGAWA. Human and rat atrial natriuretic polypeptides and their precursors. In: *Natural Products and Biological Activities*, edited by H. Imura, T. Goto, T. Murachi, and T. Nakajima. Tokyo: University of Tokyo Press, 1986, p. 319–324.

35. MCKENZIE, J. C., I. TANAKA, T. INAGAMI, K. S. MISONO, AND R. M. KLEIN. Alterations in atrial and plasma atrial natriuretic factor (ANF) content during development of hypoxia-induced pulmonary hypertension in rat. *Proc. Soc. Exp. Biol. Med.* 181: 459–463, 1986.

36. MCKENZIE, J. C., I. TANAKA, K. S. MISONO, AND T. INAGAMI. Immunocytochemical localization of atrial natriuretic factor in the kidney, adrenal medulla, pituitary and atrium of rat. Evidence for sites of action. *J. Histochem. Cytochem.* 33: 828–832, 1985.

37. MISONO, K. S., H. FUKUMI, R. T. GRAMMER, AND T. INAGAMI. Rat atrial natriuretic factor: complete amino acid sequence and disulfide linkage essential for biological activity. *Biochem. Biophys. Res. Commun.* 119: 524–529, 1984.

38. MISONO, K. S., R. T. GRAMMER, H. FUKUMI, AND T. INAGAMI. Rat atrial natriuretic factor: isolation, structure and biological activities of four major peptides. *Biochem. Biophys. Res. Commun.* 123: 444–451, 1984.

39. MIYATA, A., K. KANGAWA, T. TOSHIMORI, T. HATOH, AND H. MATSUO. Molecular forms of atrial natriuretic polypeptides in mammalian tissue and plasma. *Biochem. Biophys. Res. Commun.* 129: 248–255, 1985.

40. MIYATA, A., K. KANGAWA, T. TOSHIMORI, H. MASUDA, T. HATOH, AND H. MATSUO. Molecular forms and distribution of atrial natriuretic polypeptide (ANPs) in rat tissue and plasma. In: *Peptide Chemistry 1985*, edited by Y. Kiso. Osaka, Japan: Protein Res. Found., 1986, p. 17–22.

41. MORII, N., K. NAKAO, M. KIHARA, A. SUGAWARA, M. SAKAMOTO, Y. YAMORI, AND H. IMURA. Decreased content in left atrium and increased plasma concentration of atrial natriuretic polypeptide in spontaneously hypertensive rats (SHR) and SHR stroke-prone. *Biochem. Biophys. Res. Commun.* 135: 74–81, 1986.

42. MORII, N., K. NAKAO, A. SUGAWARA, M. SAKAMOTO, M. SUDA, M. SHIMOKURA, Y. KISO, M. KIHARA, Y. YAMORI, AND H. IMURA. Occurrence of atrial natriuretic polypeptide in brain. *Biochem. Biophys. Res. Commun.* 127: 413–419, 1985.

43. NAKAMURA, M., G. KATSUURA, K. NAKAO, AND H. IMURA. Antidipsogenic action of alpha-human natriuretic polypeptide administered intracerebroventricularly in rats. *Neurosci. Lett.* 58: 1–6, 1985.

44. NAKAMARU, M., R. TAKAYANAGI, AND T. INAGAMI. Effect of atrial natriuretic factor on central antiogensin II-induced responses in rats. *Peptides Fayetteville* 7: 373–375, 1986.

45. NAKAO, K., A. SUGAWARA, N. MORII, M. SAKAMOTO, M. SUDA, J. SONEDA, T. BAN, M. KIHARA, Y. YAMORI, M. SHIMOKURA, Y. KISO, AND H. IMURA. Radioimmunoassay for α-human and rat atrial natriuretic polypeptide. *Biochem. Biophys. Res. Commun.* 124: 815–821, 1984.

46. NAKAOKA, H., K. IMATAKA, M. AMANO, J. FUJII, M. ISHIBASHI, AND T. YAMAJI. Plasma levels of atrial natriuretic factor in patients with congestive heart failure. *N. Engl. J. Med.* 313: 892–893, 1985.

47. NAKAYAMA, K., H. OHKUBO, T. HIROSE, S. INAYAMA, AND S. NAKANISHI. mRNA sequence for human cardiodilatin-atrial natriuretic factor precursor and regulation of precursor mRNA in rat atria. *Nature Lond.* 310: 699–701, 1984.

48. NARUSE, K., M. NARUSE, K. OBANA, F. KURIMOTO, H. SAKURAI, T. HONDA, H. DEMURA, T. INAGAMI, AND K. SHIZUME. Plasma immunoreactive alpha-human atrial natriuretic polypeptide in patients with disorders of blood pressure and body fluid. *Peptides Fayetteville* 7: 141–145, 1986.

49. OBANA, K., M. NARUSE, T. INAGAMI, A. B. BROWN, K. NARUSE, F. KURIMOTO, H. SAKURAI, H. DEMURA, AND K. SHIZUME. Atrial natriuretic factor inhibits vasopressin secretion from rat posterior pituitary. *Biochem. Biophys. Res. Commun.* 132: 1088–1094, 1985.

50. OIKAWA, S., M. IMAI, A. UENO, S. TANAKA, T. NOGUCHI, H. NAKAZATO, K. KANGAWA, A. FUKUDA, AND H. MATSUO. Cloning and sequence analysis of cDNA encoding a precursor for human atrial natriuretic polypeptide. *Nature Lond.* 309: 724–726, 1984.

51. RAINE, A. E. G., F. B. MÜLLER, R. M. L. BROUWER, E. BÜRGISSER, P. BOLLI, AND F. R. BÜHLER. Plasma atrial natriuretic factor in man: parallel change with renin, noradrenaline and salt balance (abstr.). *Hypertension Dallas* 7: 838, 1985.

52. RODEHEFFER, R. J., I. TANAKA, T. IMADA, A. HOLLISTER, AND T. INAGAMI. Secretion of atrial natriuretic factor into human central circulation. *J. Am. Coll. Cardiol.* 8: 18–26, 1986.

53. SAGNELLA, G. A., N. D. MARKANDU, A. C. SHORE, AND G. A. McGREGOR. Effects of changes in dietary sodium intake and saline infusion on immunoreactive atrial natriuretic peptide in human plasma. *Lancet* 2: 1206–1211, 1985.

54. SAGNELLA, G. A., N. D. MARKANDU, A. C. SHORE, AND G. A. McGREGOR. Raised circulating levels of atrial natriuretic peptide in essential hypertension. *Lancet* 1: 179–181, 1986.

55. SAMSON, W. K. Atrial natriuretic factor inhibits dehydration and hemorrhage-induced vasopressin release. *Neuroendocrinology* 40: 277–279, 1985.

56. SAMSON, W. K. Dehydration-induced alterations in rat brain vasopressin and atrial natriuretic factor immunoreactivity. *Endocrinology* 117: 1279–1281, 1985.

57. SAPER, C. B., D. G. STANDAERT, M. G. CURRIE, D. SCHWARTZ, D. M. GELLER, AND P. NEEDLEMAN. Atriopeptin-immunoreactive neurons in the brain: presence in cardiovascular regulatory areas. *Science Wash. DC* 227: 1047–1049, 1985.

58. SCHWARTZ, D., D. M. GELLER, P. T. MANNING, N. R. SIEGEL, K. F. FOK, C. E. SMITH, AND P. NEEDLEMAN. Ser-Leu-Arg-Arg-atriopeptin III: the major circulating form of atrial peptide. *Science Wash. DC* 229: 397–400, 1985.

59. SEIDMAN, C. E., A. D. DUBY, E. CHOI, R. M. GRAHAM, E. HABER, C. HOMCY, J. A. SMITH, AND J. G. SEIDMAN. The structure of rat preproatrial natriuretic factor as defined by a complementary DNA clone. *Science Wash. DC* 225: 324–326, 1984.

60. SHIBASAKI, T., M. NARUSE, A. MASUDA, Y. S. KIM, T. IMAKI, N. YAMAUCHI, H. DEMURA, T. INAGAMI, AND K. SHIZUME. Atrial natriuretic factor is released from rat hypothalamus in vitro. *Biochem. Biophys. Res. Commun.* 136: 590–595, 1986.

61. SHIBASAKI, T., M. NARUSE, N. YAMAUCHI, A. MASUDA, T. IMAKI, K. NARUSE, H. DEMURA, N. LING, T. INAGAMI, AND K. SHIZUME. Rat atrial natriuretic factor suppresses proopiomelanocortin-derived peptides secretion from both anterior and intermediate lobe cells and growth hormone release from anterior lobe cells of rat pituitary in vivo. *Biochem. Biophys. Res. Commun.* 135: 1035–1041, 1986.

62. SHIONO, S., K. NAKAO, N. MORII, T. YAMADA, H. ITOH, M. SAKAMOTO, A. SUGAWARA, Y. SAITO, G. KATSUURA, AND H. IMURA. Nature of atrial natriuretic polypeptide in rat brain. *Biochem. Biophys. Res. Commun.* 135: 728–734, 1986.

63. STONE, R. A., AND C. C. GLEMBOTSKI. Immunoreactive atrial natriuretic peptide in the rat eye: molecular forms in anterior uvea and retina. *Biochem. Biophys. Res. Commun.* 134: 1022–1028, 1986.

64. SUGAWARA, A., K. NAKAO, N. MORII, M. SAKAMOTO, M. SUDA, M. SHIMOKURA, Y. KISO, M. KIHARA, Y. YAMORI, K. NISHIMURA, J. SONEDA, T. BAN, AND H. IMURA. Alpha-human atrial natriuretic polypeptide is released from the heart and circulates in the body. *Biochem. Biophys. Res. Commun.* 129: 439–446, 1985.

65. SUGIYAMA, M., H. FUKUMI, R. T. GRAMMER, K. S. MISONO, Y. YABE, Y. MORISAWA, AND T. INAGAMI. Synthesis of atrial natriuretic peptides and studies on structural factors in tissue specificity. *Biochem. Biophys. Res. Commun.* 123: 338–344, 1984.

66. TAKAYANAGI, R., T. IMADA, AND T. INAGAMI. Synthesis and presence of atrial natriuretic factor in rat ventricle. *Biochem. Biophys. Res. Commun.* In press.

67. TANAKA, I., AND T. INAGAMI. Increased concentration of plasma immunoreactive ANF in Dahl salt sensitive rats with sodium chloride-induced hypertension. *J. Hypertens.* 4: 109–112, 1986.

68. TANAKA, I., AND T. INAGAMI. Release of immunoreactive atrial natriuretic factor from rat hypothalamus in vitro. *Eur. J. Pharmacol.* 122: 353–355, 1986.

69. TANAKA, I., K. MISONO, AND T. INAGAMI. Atrial natriuretic factor in rat hypothalamus, atria and plasma: determination by specific radioimmunoassay. *Biochem. Biophys. Res. Commun.* 124: 663–668, 1984.

70. THIBAULT, G., R. GARCIA, M. CANTIN, J. GENEST, C. LAZURE, N. G. SEIDAH, AND M. CHRÉTIEN. Primary structure of a high Mr form of rat atrial natriuretic factor. *FEBS Lett.* 167: 352–356, 1984.

71. THIBAULT, G., C. LAZURE, E. L. SCHIFFRIN, J. GUTKOWSKA, L. CHARTIER, R. GARCIA, N. G. SEIDAH, M. CHRÉTIEN, J. GENEST, AND M. CANTIN. Identification of a biologically active circulating form of rat atrial natriuretic factor. *Biochem. Biophys. Res. Commun.* 130: 981–986, 1985.

72. TIKKANEN, I., F. FYHRQUIST, K. METSÄRINNE, AND R. LEIDENIUS. Plasma atrial natriuretic peptide in cardiac disease and during infusion in healthy volunteers. *Lancet* 2: 66–69, 1985.

73. VUOLTEENAHO, O., O. ARJAMAA, AND N. LING. Atrial natriuretic polypeptides (ANP): rat atria store high molecular weight precursor but secrete processed peptides of 25–35 amino acids. *Biochem. Biophys. Res. Commun.* 129: 82–88, 1985.
74. YAMAJI, T., M. ISHIBASHI, H. NAKAOKA, K. IMATAKA, M. AMANO, AND J. FUJII. Possible role for atrial natriuretic peptide in polyuria associated with paroxysmal atrial arrhythmias (letter to the editor). *Lancet* 1: 1211, 1985.
75. YAMANAKA, M., B. GREENBERG, L. JOHNSON, J. SEILHAMER, M. BREWER, T. FRIEDEMANN, J. MILLER, S. ATLAS, J. LARAGH, J. LEWICKI, AND J. FIDDES. Cloning and sequence analysis of the cDNA for the rat atrial natriuretic factor precursor. *Nature Lond.* 309: 719–722, 1984.
76. YANDLE, T. G., I. CROZIER, E. A. ESPINER, H. IKRAM, AND M. G. NICHOLS. Production, plasma levels and clearance of atrial natriuretic peptide in man (abstr.). *Hypertension Dallas* 7: 838, 1985.
77. YOSHINAGA, K., K. YAMAGUCHI, K. ABE, Y. MIYAKE, K. OTSUBO, S. HORI, H. OONO, A. KANAI, K. MARUNO, AND Y. MISHIMA. Determination of atrial natriuretic polypeptide (ANP) in human plasma. *Biomed. Res.* 7: 173–179, 1986.
78. ZAMIR, N., G. SKOFITSCH, R. L. ESDAY, AND D. M. JACOBOWITZ. Distribution of immunoreactive atrial natriuretic peptide in the central nervous system of the rat. *Brain Res.* 365: 105–111, 1986.

6

Physiological Actions of Atrial Natriuretic Factor

STEVEN A. ATLAS AND JOHN H. LARAGH

Cardiovascular Center and the Department of Medicine, Cornell University Medical College, New York, New York

ATRIAL NATRIURETIC FACTOR (ANF) is a recently discovered polypeptide hormone that is synthesized and stored in atrial muscle cells (9, 21, 31, 32, 71, 79). There is evidence that lower levels of ANF are synthesized in several other tissues, including ventricle and brain, but it is presumed that the atrium is the principal source of circulating ANF in mammals. It has been known for nearly 30 years that atrial muscle cells contain secretory granules and a well-developed Golgi apparatus, as found in other hormone-secreting cells (59, 63); such granules are not present in the mammalian ventricle but are present in ventricle and atrium in lower vertebrates (12). Work done in the 1970s suggested that alterations in fluid and electrolyte balance were associated with changes in the density of the atrial granules (29, 75). In 1981 de Bold and co-workers (32) demonstrated that extracts of rat atrium contained a factor that induces a marked increase in sodium excretion when administered to intact rats; subsequent work showed that this factor is associated with the atrial granules (22, 30, 44). More recently it has been shown that ANF comprises a number of structurally related small peptides derived from a 126–amino acid residue precursor (10, 28, 42, 61, 62, 73, 76, 82, 99, 100, 123). The numerous peptides isolated from atrium, ranging between 21 and 35 amino acid residues, probably resulted in large part from nonspecific proteolysis of the precursor during extraction and purification procedures. Although the precursor is the major storage form in atrium (41), it appears that a 28-residue peptide is the major circulating form (38, 42, 61, 98, 110, 122). Plasma levels of immunoreactive ANF under basal conditions are reported to be on the order of 10^{-12}–10^{-11} M in unanesthetized animals and humans (25, 38, 68, 70, 102, 109, 122).

In addition to inducing natriuresis and diuresis, ANF has several actions of potential physiological significance that have been demonstrated in vitro or by administration of the peptide to intact animals. These actions include inhibitory effects on steroidogenesis, most prominently affecting aldosterone biosynthesis, and on the secretion of renin, vasopressin, and possibly ACTH; behavioral effects on thirst and salt appetite; a relaxant effect on contracted vascular smooth muscle; effects on systemic hemodynamics and intravascular volume regulation that may lead to a reduction in blood pressure; and complex renal hemodynamic effects, including an increase in glomerular filtration rate (GFR), which apparently play an important role in its natriuretic and renin-suppressing actions.

Membrane-bound receptors for ANF have been identified on all its potential target tissues; although its exact mechanisms of action remain to be defined, the peptide has been shown to have effects on known cellular intermediates. By activating the particulate (membrane-bound) form of guanylate cyclase, ANF causes striking increases in tissue levels of cGMP (52, 117). In fact, ANF is the only substance of mammalian origin that has been shown to activate this enzyme. In certain target tissues, ANF has also been shown to inhibit adenylate cyclase (4). While some of its actions (e.g., on vascular smooth muscle and adrenal cortex) probably depend ultimately on a reduction in cytosolic calcium, evidence of this has yet to be provided.

This chapter provides an overview of the actions of ANF that may be relevant to the physiological regulation of fluid and electrolyte balance and cardiovascular homeostasis. The potentially important actions of circulating ANF are emphasized, although some of the effects described may also be relevant to the existence of immunoreactive ANF–containing neurons and ANF-binding sites in hypothalamus and other brain regions (58, 87, 92, 95, 104, 109). In some cases, particularly with regard to studies in intact animal preparations, supraphysiological concentrations of the peptide have been employed to demonstrate these effects. A brief consideration of what is known about the regulation of ANF secretion will be useful to place these findings in perspective. However, in the absence of specific antagonists of ANF, only tentative conclusions can be made regarding the physiological significance of these actions.

EFFECTS ON THE KIDNEY

Renal Hemodynamic Actions

In the isolated perfused rat kidney, ANF induces a major increase in GFR accompanied by an increase in renal resistance (10, 18, 71). Increases in GFR have also been demonstrated in intact animals and humans (Fig. 1; 16, 25, 54, 71, 72, 118). The effect on GFR is independent of changes in total renal blood flow (16, 72, 79) and is probably due to an increase in glomerular capillary hydraulic pressure induced by constriction of the efferent arteriole and, possibly, dilation of the afferent arteriole (43, 55). By virtue of its vasorelaxant effect, ANF can cause net renal vasodilation when vascular tonus is markedly increased (18, 71, 84, 107). Under basal conditions in vivo, however, sustained

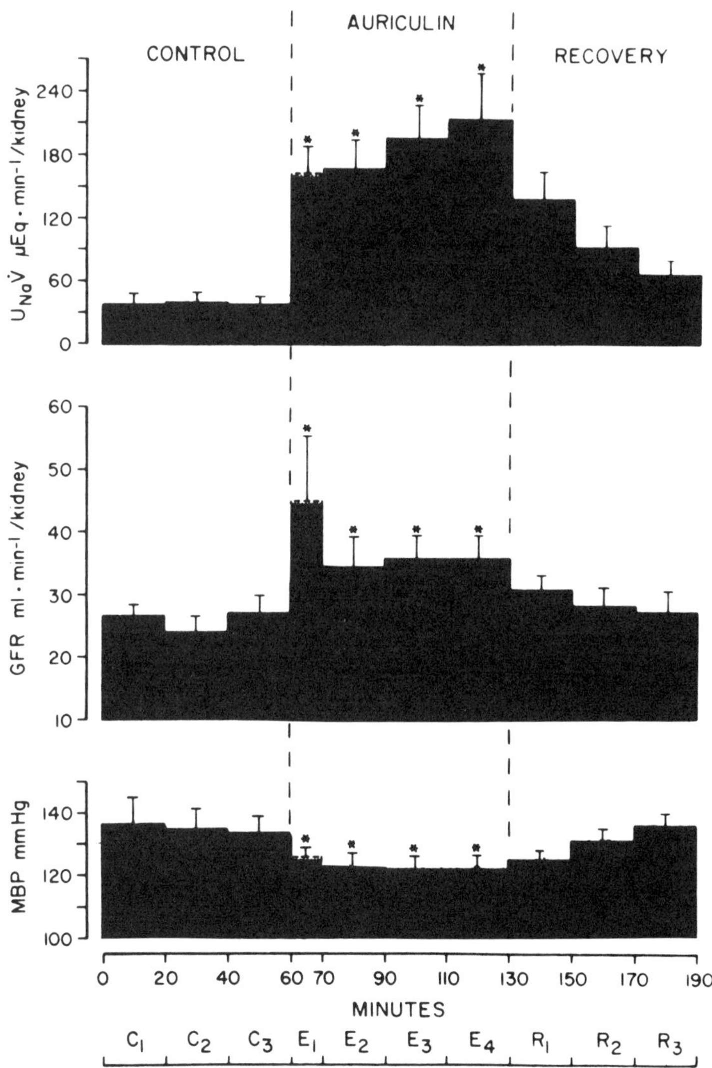

FIG. 1. Time course of effects of synthetic atrial natriuretic factor (ANF; auriculin) on mean blood pressure (MBP), glomerular filtration rate (GFR), and sodium excretion ($U_{Na}\dot{V}$) in anesthetized dogs. ANF was given as a 1.0 μg/kg prime followed by constant infusion of 0.1 μg·kg^{-1}·min^{-1} (40 pmol·kg^{-1}·min^{-1}). C, control; E, experimental; and R, recovery periods. Results are expressed as means ± SE ($n = 5$). * $P < 0.05$ compared with control values. [From Maack et al. (72).]

infusion of the peptide leads to only transient increases in total renal blood flow (16, 72). There is evidence, however, that ANF might cause a redistribution of blood flow to the inner medulla (15).

Effects on Renal Excretory Function

Continuous administration of synthetic ANF leads to a sustained natriuresis and diuresis together with lesser increases in calcium, magnesium, phosphate, and potassium excretion (15, 16, 25, 54, 72, 118). Increases in free-water clearance have also been demonstrated in human subjects (25, 118); evidence of this in water-loaded subjects (25) may suggest increased free-water formation in the thick ascending limb, implying that ANF increases sodium delivery to this nephron segment. This observation, together with the effects on divalent ion excretion, suggests a major action of ANF in the proximal portion of the nephron (i.e., either on GFR or on proximal reabsorption). On the other hand, the kaluresis induced by ANF is highly variable and often not sustained (25), despite a sizable and maintained natriuresis; inhibition of aldosterone release is unlikely to fully account for this observation, raising the possibility of some action beyond the distal site of Na^+-K^+-H^+ exchange.

Micropuncture experiments and studies on isolated perfused nephron segments or other isolated epithelia have not revealed a direct effect of the peptide on active sodium transport that can fully explain these effects (71); in particular, ANF has no effect on sodium reabsorption in superficial proximal tubules (54). A recent report suggests that ANF can inhibit amiloride-sensitive sodium transport in an established cell line derived from renal tubular epithelium (20). If present in the intact kidney (e.g., in the collecting duct), such an effect would likely contribute to ANF-induced natriuresis, but available evidence suggests that this mechanism is unlikely, by itself, to play a major role.

The unique renal hemodynamic actions of ANF clearly play a critical role in the full expression of ANF-induced natriuresis, since the latter can be abolished by constriction of the renal artery (17, 26, 107). Such studies, as illustrated in Figure 2, suggest an important role for ANF-induced changes in GFR; however, it is unlikely that an increase in GFR can, by itself, explain the marked increase in fractional sodium excretion produced by ANF (71). Other renal hemodynamic actions of the peptide could lead to major secondary effects on tubular reabsorption, which would disrupt glomerulotubular balance. For instance, ANF induces a washout of the medullary interstitial concentrating gradient (71), possibly due to the shift in blood flow to the medulla (15), which might also be expected to increase medullary interstitial fluid pressure. These events can have a major impact on tubular sodium reabsorption, especially in the medullary thin ascending limb of Henle's loop and/or collecting duct. Renal ANF-binding sites and ANF-induced cGMP production are observed mainly in the cortical glomeruli and, to a lesser extent, in the papilla, where they are associated with vasa recta and/or collecting duct (14, 112). From the available data, it seems likely that the renal hemodynamic

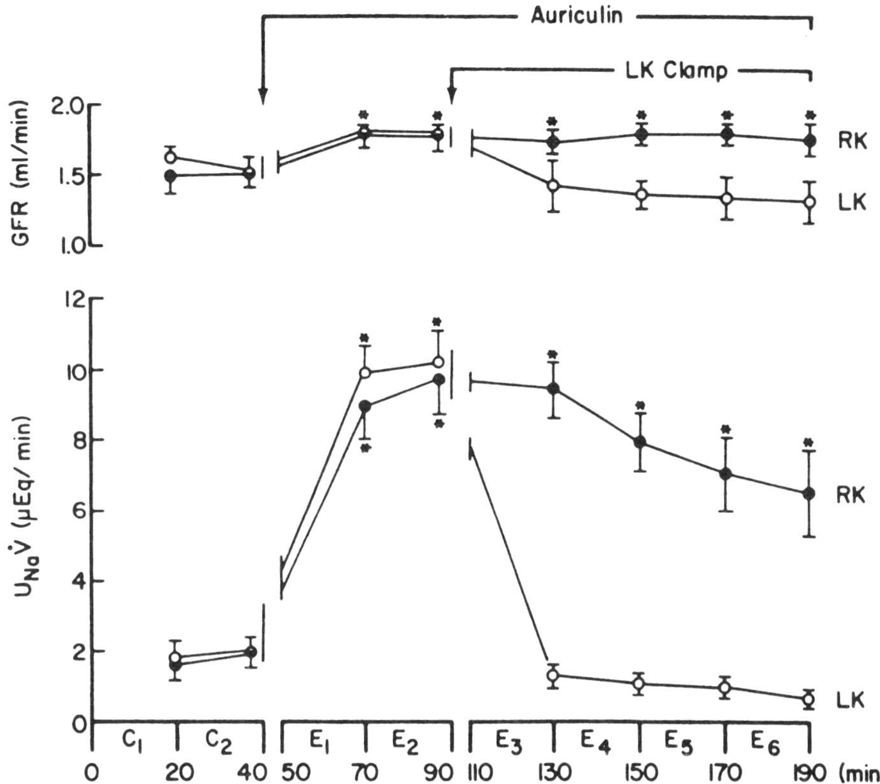

FIG. 2. Time course of effects of atrial natriuretic factor (ANF; auriculin) infusion on glomerular filtration rate (GFR) and urinary sodium excretion ($U_{Na}\dot{V}$) in right (RK) and left (LK) kidneys of anesthetized rats. ANF was administered as a constant infusion throughout experimental (E) periods. At point indicated, a late LK clamp was produced by constricting a loop placed around the aorta between right and left renal arteries until mean pressure in the femoral artery was reduced to 75–80 mmHg. This returned both GFR and $U_{Na}\dot{V}$ to control (C) levels in LK, while both responses were sustained in RK. Results are means ± SE ($n = 6$). * $P < 0.01$ vs. control. [From Camargo et al. (17).]

actions of ANF, i.e., increased GFR combined with secondary effects on tubular sodium reabsorption, play a major role in the natriuresis induced by the peptide (71).

Effects on Renin Secretion

As shown in Figure 3, ANF induces a prompt and marked inhibition of renin secretion in intact dogs (16, 72), a rather remarkable effect considering the concurrent fall in arterial pressure (see Fig. 1). A reduction in peripheral plasma renin activity has been observed in both conscious and anesthetized dogs (11, 72) and in normal human subjects (25) but has been more difficult to discern in normal rats (115). The mechanisms through which ANF acutely reduces renin secretion remain to be fully defined, but its hemodynamic effects

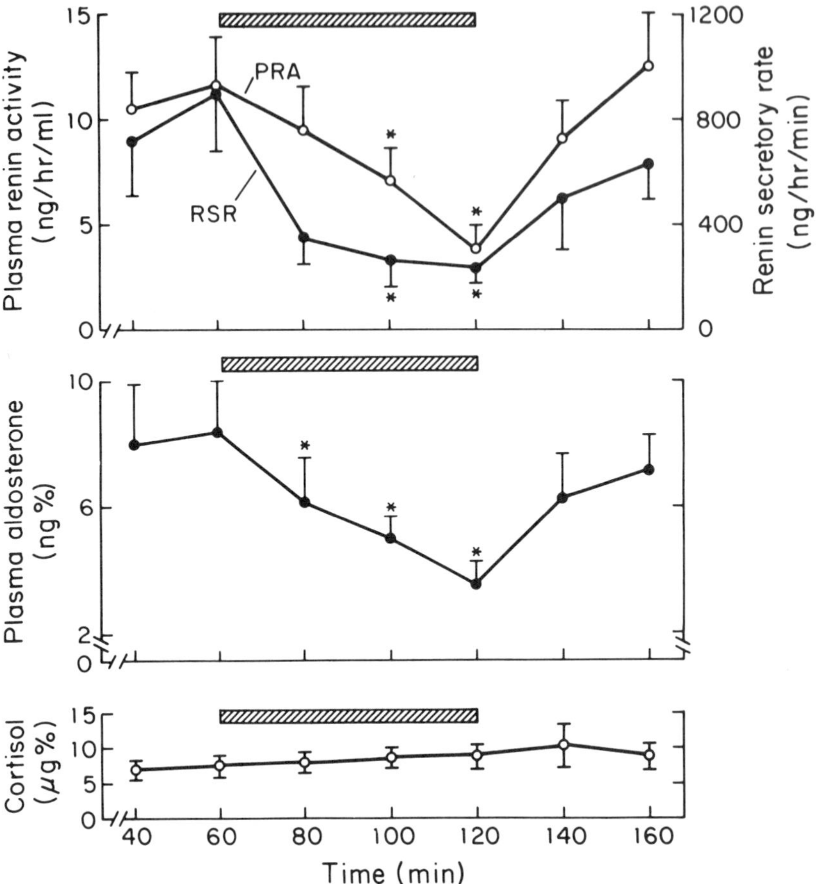

FIG. 3. Effect of synthetic ANF on renin secretory rate (RSR), plasma renin acivity (PRA), plasma aldosterone, and cortisol in anesthetized normotensive dogs. *Hatched bar*, infusion period. ANF was given as a 1.0 µg/kg prime followed by constant infusion of 0.1 $\mu g \cdot kg^{-1} \cdot min^{-1}$ (40 pmol$\cdot$ kg$^{-1}\cdot$min^{-1}). [From Maack et al. (72).]

on the kidney are likely to be involved (11, 16, 72, 108, 115). The ANF-induced increase in GFR, by increasing the filtered solute load, probably leads to increased sodium chloride delivery to the macula densa. In addition, by causing afferent arteriolar dilation, ANF might conceivably increase hydrostatic pressure along the afferent arteriole. A direct inhibitory effect of ANF on renin release by the juxtaglomerular cells is also possible, and there is a preliminary report that very large concentrations of ANF (10^{-7} M or greater) can cause slight inhibition of renin release in rat kidney slices (81). In the intact animal, however, there is evidence that renal hemodynamic changes play a critical role in allowing expression of the renin-suppressing effect of ANF. Acute constriction of one renal artery, which provokes unilateral secretion of renin from the ischemic kidney and which prevents the ANF-induced renal hemodynamic effects, completely blocks the ability of ANF to acutely reduce renin-secretion rate and peripheral plasma renin activity in the dog (108). Renin secretion actually tends to rise under these experimental conditions (Fig. 4), probably due to the further reduction in renal perfusion pressure induced by ANF. More recently it has been shown that ANF does not inhibit renin secretion in the nonfiltering kidney (83), suggesting that ANF-induced increases in distal sodium delivery are likely to play an important role under normal circumstances.

A similar finding has been observed in chronic two-kidney, one clip renovascular rats (114, 115). In these animals, which have markedly increased base-line plasma renin levels, constant infusion of ANF caused a slight but significant further increase in plasma renin activity. In the same study, however, ANF suppressed plasma renin in sodium-depleted, one-kidney, one clip rats (115). In this setting, even subtle increases in distal delivery of sodium chloride might inhibit renin secretion, since the macula densa would be expected to be exquisitely sensitive to changes in solute delivery in the sodium-depleted state. A similar mechanism might contribute to the reduction in plasma renin observed after long-term administration of ANF to two-kidney, one clip rats (46).

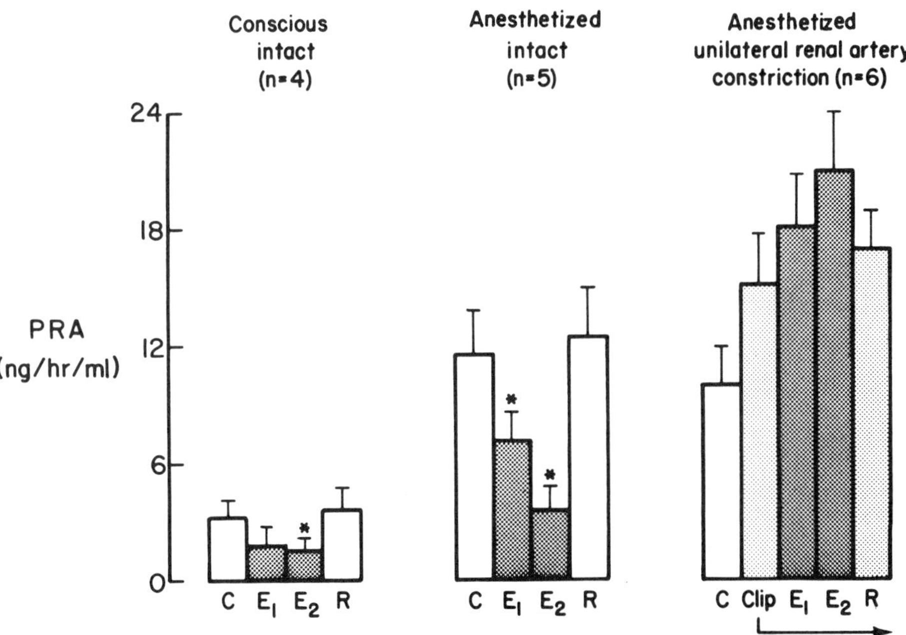

FIG. 4. Effect of synthetic ANF on plasma renin activity (PRA) in intact dogs or dogs with acute unilateral renal artery constriction. ANF was given as a 1.0 μg/kg prime followed by constant infusion of 0.1 μg·kg^{-1}·min^{-1} (40 pmol·kg^{-1}·min^{-1}). Unilateral renal artery constriction (Clip) was produced with a snare around the left renal artery that reduced renal perfusion pressure to 80–90 mmHg and prevented the ANF-induced increase in GFR; ANF infusion was begun 1 h after constriction. C, last control; E$_1$, E$_2$, experimental (40- and 60-min ANF infusion); R, last recovery periods. [From Atlas et al. (11).]

EFFECTS ON STEROIDOGENESIS

Effects on Aldosterone

It has been shown that ANF inhibits aldosterone production by rat or bovine adrenal cortical cells in vitro (8, 23, 33, 50, 67) and lowers plasma aldosterone levels in experimental animals (24, 79, 114, 115) and normal human subjects (25). The peptide inhibits basal aldosterone production by isolated bovine and rat adrenal zona glomerulosa cells and also antagonizes the stimulation of aldosterone by agonists such as angiotensin II (8, 23, 24, 33, 50, 67), ACTH (24, 33, 67), dibutyryl cAMP (50), and potassium (24, 50). Although ANF thus has generic actions on the adrenal glomerulosa, there is evidence for some preferential effect on angiotensin II–stimulated steroidogenesis, since angiotensin II, unlike other agonists, is unable to overcome the inhibitory effect of ANF on aldosterone production by isolated rat glomerulosa (7). The inhibitory action is exerted principally at the early portion of the steroidogenic pathway, at some point prior to mitochondrial cholesterol uptake and side-chain cleavage (50); an effect on the distal portion of the aldosterone biosynthetic pathway has also been reported in angiotensin-stimulated cells (19).

In the intact dog and normal humans, ANF-induced reduction in plasma aldosterone concentration occurs in association with a fall in plasma renin activity (see Fig. 3; 25, 72). Thus the aldosterone-suppressing effect could be in part secondary to the presumed concurrent fall in plasma angiotensin II. There is evidence, however, that ANF can directly inhibit aldosterone production in vivo, since its effects on renin and aldosterone can be dissociated in certain circumstances (11, 25, 108, 114, 115). For instance, ANF is still able to lower plasma aldosterone significantly in dogs in which a fall in renin is prevented by unilateral renal artery constriction (108). An even more dramatic effect is observed in renin-dependent, two-kidney, one clip hypertensive rats, in which ANF induces profound reductions in plasma aldosterone (114, 115), despite concurrent increases in plasma renin activity (Fig. 5). This finding,

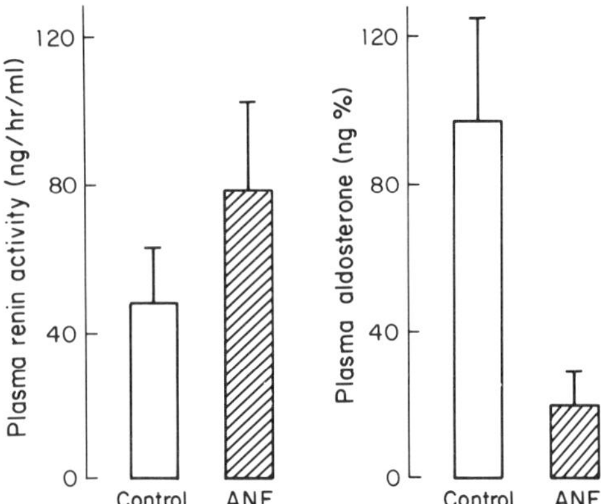

FIG. 5. Effect of synthetic ANF on plasma renin activity (PRA) and plasma aldosterone in conscious, unrestrained two-kidney, one clip Goldblatt hypertensive rats ($n = 5$). Blood samples were obtained just before (Control) and after 60 min (ANF) of constant infusion (120 pmol·kg^{-1}·min^{-1}). ANF caused a significant fall in plasma aldosterone ($P < 0.001$) despite concurrent increase in renin ($P < 0.05$). [From Atlas et al. (11).]

together with other evidence (7, 24), emphasizes the potency of ANF as an antagonist of the adrenal actions of angiotensin II. In addition, in patients with congestive heart failure, ANF infusion causes a major decrease in plasma aldosterone concentration, despite the fact that its ability to inhibit renin secretion (or to induce natriuresis) is severely blunted (25).

Although it is clear that ANF-induced inhibition of aldosterone secretion does not contribute to its acute natriuretic action (which is evident within seconds of beginning the infusion), the impact of this effect on long-term fluid volume regulation is obviously of major potential importance.

Effects on Glucocorticoids

The fact that ANF acts early in the steroid biosynthetic pathway suggests that it could potentially affect production of other steroid hormones. The specificity of its action therefore probably lies in the distribution of specific binding sites. In some species, the effect of ANF appears to be specific for aldosterone production by the zona glomerulosa. There is no effect on corticosterone production by isolated rat fasciculata-reticularis cells (8, 67), and ANF receptors are located mainly in the zona glomerulosa in this species (14). Infusion of ANF also has no effect on plasma cortisol in intact dogs (see Fig. 3; 72). This peptide has, however, been shown to decrease cortisol production by bovine adrenal cells (33), consistent with the presence of receptors in all zones of bovine adrenal cortex. Infusion of ANF also tends to depress plasma cortisol slightly in humans (25). Although the latter observation might, by analogy, be attributable to a direct effect on the inner cortical zones, an indirect effect, via ACTH suppression, must also be considered.

Effects on Gonadal Steroids

It has been shown that ANF activates particulate guanylate cyclase in rat testis, among other tissues (117). A recent report indicates that ANF causes accumulation of cGMP and marked inhibition of adenylate cyclase in cultured mouse Leydig tumor cells (85), together with slight inhibition of progesterone production by these cells; striking effects on cyclic nucleotides were noted under basal conditions, whereas inhibition of steroidogenesis could only be detected in luteinizing hormone– or human chorionic gonadotropin–stimulated cells (85). In contrast to these findings, there is also a report that ANF can increase basal testosterone production by mouse interstitial cells (13). There are as yet no reports demonstrating an effect on testicular (or ovarian) steroid production in intact animals.

EFFECTS ON PITUITARY HORMONE SECRETION

Vasopressin

Systemically administered ANF has been shown to have a potent inhibitory effect on hemorrhage- or dehydration-induced vasopressin release in intact rats (91). Furthermore, injection of ANF into the third ventricle inhibits vasopressin release even under basal conditions (93). Although the locus of action of ANF is unclear, a direct effect on the posterior pituitary is possible, since ANF decreases vasopressin release from the isolated rat neurohypophysis stimulated by K^+ depolarization in vitro (21). In the same preparation, however, ANF by itself stimulated vasopressin release (21, 60), an effect that has not been demonstrated in intact animals. A more recent study, using superfused neurohypophyseal fragments, has shown that 10^{-10} M ANF can inhibit basal vasopressin release and also partially block stimulation of release induced by either KCl or angiotensin II (80).

Anterior Pituitary Hormones

Infusion of ANF tends to decrease plasma cortisol in humans. More impressive is the striking rebound increase in plasma cortisol after cessation of ANF infusion (25). Because ANF infusion produces systemic hemodynamic effects that might normally be expected to provoke ACTH release, a possible explanation for the observed pattern of cortisol response might be that a rise in ACTH release is prevented by ANF but occurs promptly when the infusion is stopped.

Inhibition of adenylate cyclase by ANF has been demonstrated in anterior pituitary (3). A recent study suggests that physiological concentrations of ANF inhibit release of ACTH and other pro-opiomelanocortin–derived peptides (β-endorphin and γ–melanocyte-stimulating hormone) from primary cultures of rat anterior pituitary cells (103). Lesser effects were observed on antagonism of ACTH release induced by corticotropin-releasing factor or on release of pro-opiomelanocortin–derived peptides from the intermediate lobe. In contrast, an effect on ACTH release could not be demonstrated in another recent report employing similar techniques (53).

Discrepant results concerning growth hormone release were also described in these two reports; one study showed that relatively high concentrations of ANF (10^{-9} M or greater) cause slight inhibition of basal growth hormone release or of growth hormone release stimulated by growth hormone–releasing factor (103); the other study showed no effect (53). Effects on the release of gonadotropins or other glycoprotein hormones have not been described.

There are no reports of the effects of either peripherally or centrally administered ANF on plasma levels of the anterior pituitary hormones in intact animals. Further investigation is needed to resolve the contradictory findings that have been reported with in vitro systems.

EFFECTS ON VASCULAR TISSUE

Smooth Muscle Relaxation

Several investigators have shown that ANF induces relaxation of isolated blood vessels that are precontracted with a variety of hormonal and nonhormonal agonists (27, 34, 51, 64, 119). Relaxation of nonvascular smooth muscle (e.g., the carbachol-contracted chick rectum) has also been reported (27). The vasorelaxant effect appears to be due to a direct effect on vascular smooth muscle, since the presence of an intact endothelial lining is not required (120). The mechanism of action of ANF on vessels may resemble that of the nitrate vasodilators, which stimulate cGMP formation by activating soluble (cytosolic) guanylate cyclase. For reasons that are not clear, ANF appears to exert especially pronounced antagonism toward angiotensisn II–induced vasoconstriction in vitro (Fig. 6), since increasing concentrations of this agonist are unable to overcome the relaxant effect of ANF (64).

This vasorelaxant effect has been characterized in studies employing isolated large and medium-sized arteries; direct demonstration of an effect on resistance vessels has not been reported. Nonetheless, increases in regional blood flow have been reported to occur, at least transiently, in several vascular beds, most notably the kidney (45, 57, 72, 84). Such effects have been most pronounced after bolus injections of the peptide and have generally been difficult to discern during continuous infusions in intact animals, probably because of the complex systemic hemodynamic effects induced by ANF. There is abundant evidence, both in vitro and in vivo, that the ability of ANF to produce net vasorelaxation is highly dependent on the underlying tonus of vascular smooth muscle (18, 108).

Possible Effects on Vascular Endothelium

The ANF-induced vasorelaxation does not depend on an intact endothelium. It has been shown, however, that cultured vascular endothelial cells have

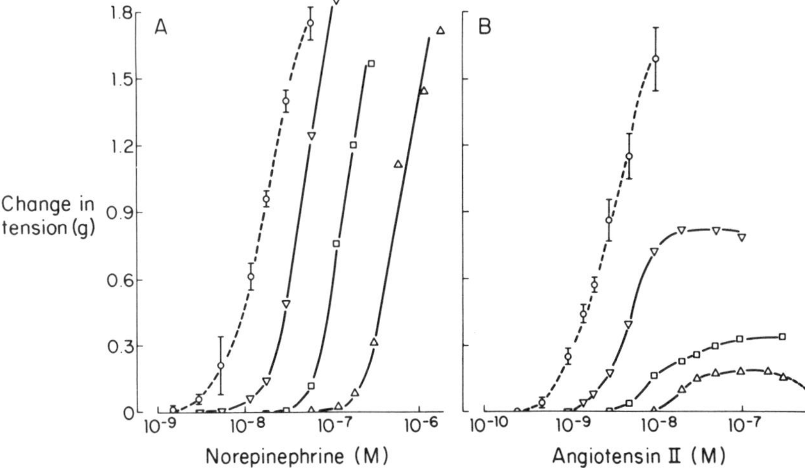

FIG. 6. Inhibition of norepinephrine-induced (*A*) and angiotensin II–induced (*B*) contraction of isolated rabbit thoracic aortic rings by increasing concentrations of ANF. *Curves,* increases in tension caused by increasing concentrations of vasoconstrictor (norepinephrine or angiotensin II). ○, Control rings; ▽, □, △, increasing concentrations of partially purified ANF added to the bath. [From Atlas (9).]

high-affinity binding sites for ANF and respond to the peptide by a marked stimulation of cGMP (97). Moreover, endothelial binding sites are prominently labeled in autoradiographic studies in the intact animal (14).

The functional counterpart, if any, to these findings is unknown. Note, however, that ANF infusion has been found to produce marked hemoconcentration, increasing both hematocrit (25, 32, 72, 118) and serum protein concentration (25) far more than would be expected on the basis of the induced renal fluid losses. A recent report indicates that this effect, together with a decrease in plasma volume, is also observed in bilaterally nephrectomized rats (2). Thus ANF appears to induce a major shift of fluid from the vascular to the extravascular space. Although the rise in serum protein concentration suggests that this might be brought about by an alteration in other Starling forces (e.g., an increase in transcapillary hydrostatic pressure), it is also conceivable that ANF could induce a selective increase in capillary hydraulic permeability by an effect on the endothelial lining (2).

SYSTEMIC HEMODYNAMIC EFFECTS

A depressor response to injection of atrial extracts was noted by de Bold and co-workers in their initial report (32); this effect has been confirmed with synthetic ANF peptides in both conscious and anesthetized normotensive and hypertensive animals (46, 65, 69, 72, 86, 101, 106, 114–116) and in humans (25, 89, 118). There is evidence that the magnitude of the depressor response to ANF differs among various hypertensive models. As shown in Figure 7, the acute blood pressure response to ANF is greater in renin-dependent, two-kidney, one clip renovascular hypertensive rats than in non-renin-dependent, one-kidney, one clip rats (115). In the latter model, prior sodium depletion,

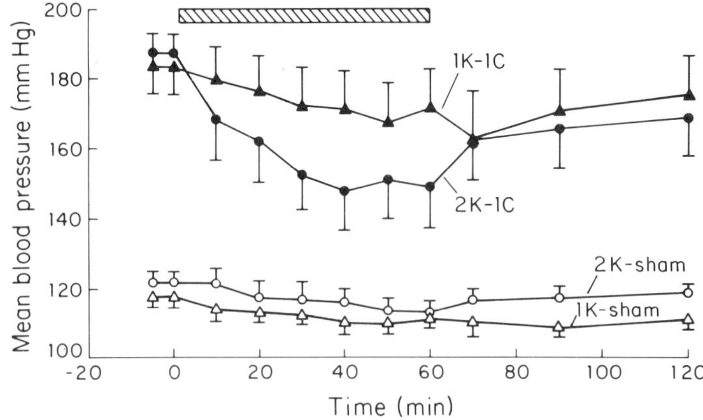

FIG. 7. Effect of synthetic ANF on blood pressure in renovascular hypertensive and sham-operated rats. *Hatched bar,* period of ANF infusion (120 pmol·kg^{-1}·min^{-1}). 1K-1C, one-kidney, one clip rats; 2K-1C, two-kidney, one clip rats; 1K-sham, one-kidney, sham-operated rats; 2K-sham, two-kidney, sham-operated rats. Blood pressure response was significantly greater ($P <$ 0.05) in 2K-1C vs. 1K-1C at all time points during ANF infusion. [From Volpe et al. (115).]

which is known to restore renin dependency, markedly enhances the blood pressure response to ANF (115). In addition, chronic administration of ANF normalizes blood pressure in two-kidney, one clip rats (46). The antihypertensive effect of ANF in renin-dependent models may be related to the high circulating levels of angiotensin II, suggesting that ANF may antagonize angiotensin II–induced vasoconstriction in vivo. Although there are reports that ANF can cause substantial blood pressure reduction in non-renin-dependent models (69, 86, 101, 106), there is evidence that the dose of ANF administered can affect not only the magnitude of the blood pressure response but also the pattern of associated hemodynamic effects (116).

In view of the known vasorelaxant effect of ANF, it was assumed initially that the depressor response to the peptide was due to a fall in vascular resistance. Transient decreases in systemic resistance have been demonstrated in anesthetized rats, particularly after bolus administration of ANF (1, 86). The available data, however, suggest that the sustained fall in arterial pressure induced by pharmacological doses of ANF, both in normotensive animals and humans and in many hypertensive models, is largely attributable to a fall in cardiac output (1, 25, 65, 69, 96, 116). In normal human subjects, ANF can induce a sizable fall in pulmonary capillary wedge pressure, even without a net reduction in arterial pressure (25), suggesting that preload effects likely contribute to the fall in cardiac output. This could be accounted for by an increase in venous capacitance or by intravascular volume contraction induced, for instance, by a fluid compartment shift. Also, ANF might indirectly affect cardiac contractility; an interaction of ANF with neural reflex mechanisms is suggested by the notable lack of reflex tachycardia, even when blood pressure is profoundly reduced (69, 115, 116), and it has also been shown that vagotomy attenuates the hypotensive action of crude atrial extracts (96). Whatever the exact mechanism, it is clear that the antihypertensive effect of sustained ANF infusion described in many studies, particularly in spontaneously hypertensive (69) and deoxycorticosterone-salt (116) rats, is due to a fall in cardiac output associated with increases in both regional and systemic vascular resistance (Fig. 8). Because of the doses of ANF employed, it is reasonable to ascribe these actions to a pharmacological effect of the peptide.

The study illustrated in Figure 8 suggests, however, that relatively low rates of ANF infusion can reduce systemic vascular resistance (without changes in cardiac output) in two-kidney, one clip hypertensive rats (116). It thus is possible that ANF, at plasma levels encountered in physiological or pathological states, could play a significant role in the regulation of arterial pressure by opposing the vasoconstrictor action of agonists such as angiotensin II.

ANTAGONISM OF HORMONE ACTION

Although ANF has undisputed direct actions (e.g., on the kidney), its effect on many target organs can be characterized as functional antagonism

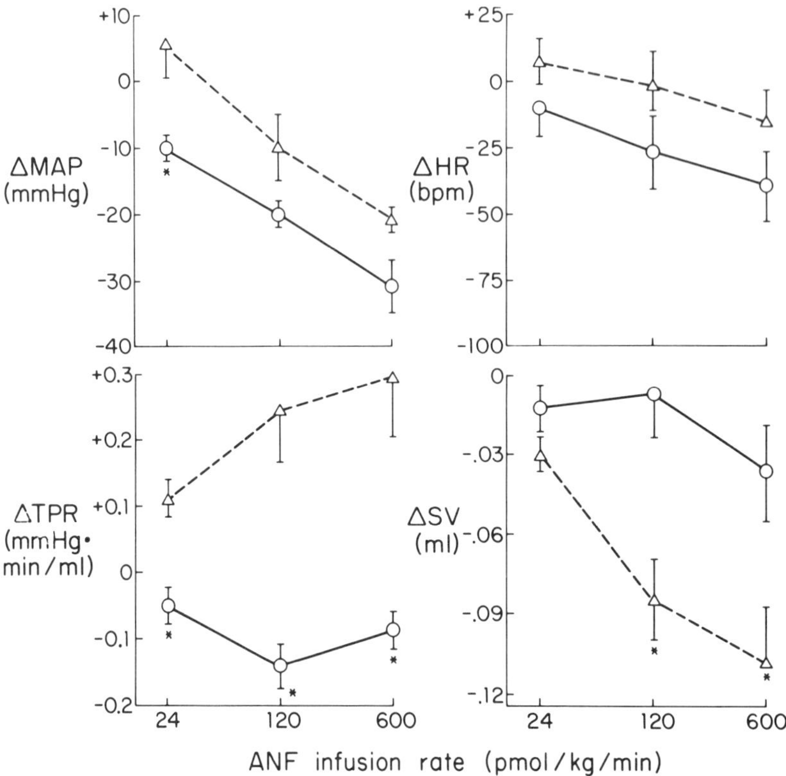

FIG. 8. Comparison of hemodynamic responses to atrial natriuretic factor (ANF) in anesthetized two-kidney, one clip (o——o) ($n = 7$) and deoxycorticosterone-salt treated (Δ– – – –Δ) ($n = 6$) hypertensive rats. Synthetic ANF was administered by graded constant infusion (30 min per dose), and the data (means ± SE) are expressed as the steady-state change in each parameter from control values. MAP, mean arterial pressure; TPR, total peripheral resistance; HR, heart rate; SV, stroke volume. * $P < 0.05$, two-kidney, one clip vs. deoxycorticosterone-salt rats. [From Volpe et al. (116).]

of the actions of hormonal agonists. This is particularly evident with regard to its actions on vascular smooth muscle, where ANF opposes vasoconstriction induced by catecholamines and other biogenic amines, angiotensin II, and vasopressin; on the adrenal cortex, where ANF inhibits aldosterone production stimulated by all known secretagogues; and in cultured testicular cells, where the reported inhibition of steroidogenesis is evident only in gonadotropin-stimulated cells. Where available, findings in the intact animal support this view of ANF as a functional antagonist, since its inhibitory effects are far more pronounced under stimulated, compared with basal, conditions; this is especially notable with regard to its effects on vascular resistance. Although there are findings that suggest a particularly prominent antagonism of the vascular and adrenal actions of angiotensin II, clarification of the physiological significance of such selectivity is needed.

The functional antagonism of angiotensin and vasopressin seem particularly relevant because ANF also has the potential to block formation or secretion of these peptides (i.e., by inhibiting renin release and by directly affecting vasopressin secretion). Furthermore, ANF has been shown to oppose other actions of these peptides: it inhibits water intake induced by centrally administered angiotensin II (5, 77), inhibits angiotensin II–stimulated vasopressin release in vitro (80), and inhibits vasopressin- or vasotocin-stimulated epithelial water transport in vitro (37, 94).

These considerations suggest that ANF may be a counter-regulatory hormone in the control of fluid volume and cardiovascular homeostasis, perhaps analogous to the roles of glucagon and calcitonin in carbohydrate and calcium metabolism. Although this admittedly arbitrary comparison might imply a relatively secondary role of ANF, such a conclusion cannot be drawn at present.

OTHER CENTRAL EFFECTS

The distribution of immunoreactive ANF–containing neurons in the hypothalamus and other brain regions suggests that ANF may have a neuro-transmitter and/or neuromodulatory function in the central control of fluid balance and blood pressure (58, 95, 104). This view is reinforced by the finding that dehydration selectively decreases ANF content in specific brain regions (92). The distribution of high-affinity binding sites in various brain structures (87) suggests, furthermore, that circulating, as well as central, ANF may have potentially important effects on central nervous system function.

Inhibitory effects of ANF on vasopressin secretion and on angiotensin II–induced drinking behavior, as well as possible effects on anterior pituitary function, have been described. It has also been shown that ANF inhibits dehydration-induced water intake (5, 77); this effect is induced by either central or systemic administration of the peptide (5). A recent study also demonstrates that centrally administered ANF specifically inhibits saline preference in sodium-depleted rats (6). Effects of centrally administered ANF on blood pressure or other cardiovascular parameters have not been reported.

PRESENT PERSPECTIVES

In the absence of specific antagonists of ANF, unqualified conclusions about the physiological relevance of any of the documented actions of ANF are not possible. Indirect lines of evidence point to a potentially important role in the control of renal sodium handling, at least in the short term. Resection of the atrial appendages has been employed to approximate the classic endocrine ablation experiment. In some, but not all, studies reported to date, this maneuver has been shown to blunt the natriuretic response to acute volume expansion (66, 113). A recent report also indicates that administration of ANF antisera to intact anesthetized rats leads to a transient decrease in sodium excretion and a rise in plasma renin activity (78).

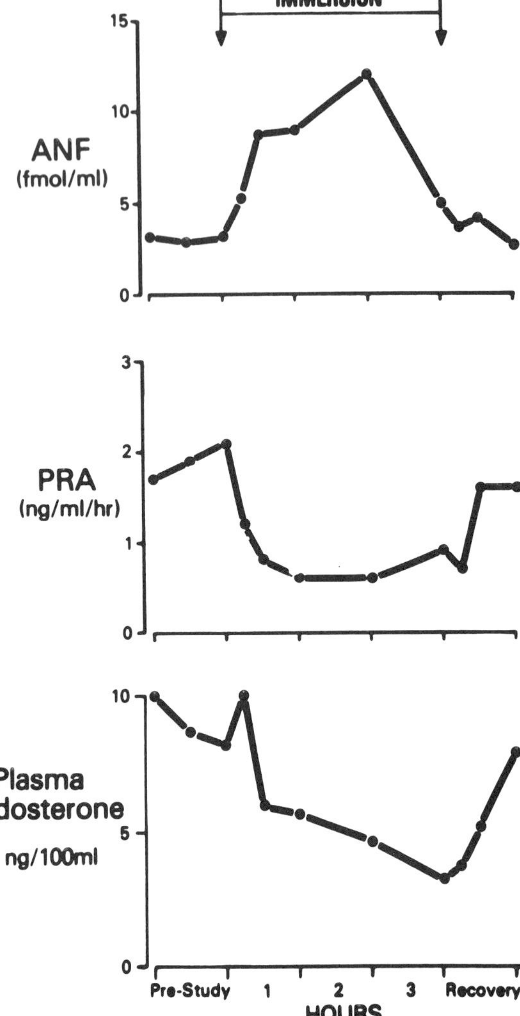

FIG. 9. Effect of water immersion to the neck on plasma ANF, plasma renin activity (PRA), and plasma aldosterone in a normal male subject. Subject remained seated throughout the 3-h immersion period and the 1-h control (prestudy) and recovery periods. $U_{Na}\dot{V}$ (not shown) increased from 63 μeq/min (prestudy) to 197 μeq/min by hour 3 of immersion and fell to 77 μeq/min during the recovery period. [From Epstein et al. (38).]

Available data on the factors that regulate ANF secretion tend to reinforce these findings. Several maneuvers provoke increased ANF plasma levels in vivo, including acute volume expansion (68), mechanical distension of the atria (70), infusion of pressor agents (74), and increases in central blood volume induced by water immersion to the neck (38, 39). The latter is illustrated in Figure 9. In addition, plasma levels of ANF increase transiently during induction of atrial tachyarrhythmias (121) and are chronically elevated in patients with poorly compensated congestive heart failure (25, 102, 111). In the latter condition, plasma ANF levels are frequently on the order of 10^{-10} M (25, 102), even as high as 7×10^{-10} M (S. A. Atlas, R. J. Cody, unpublished observations); such plasma concentrations unquestionably induce natriuresis, increased GFR, hemoconcentration, and decreased plasma renin and aldosterone in normal humans (25), but renal responses are likely impaired in heart failure due to poor renal perfusion (11, 17, 25, 26, 107).

The common thread among the experimental and clinical conditions associated with elevations of plasma ANF is an increase in the degree of atrial stretch or wall tension, a mechanism for acute ANF release that has also been elicited in isolated heart preparations (36). It appears that ANF exits the heart mainly via the coronary sinus (40), suggesting that ANF secreted by right and left atria are released together. It seems likely, nonetheless, that various provocative factors might differentially affect synthesis and/or secretion by the two atria. For instance, it is tempting to speculate that factors increasing preload to the heart might affect right atrial secretion, whereas factors increasing cardiac afterload might predominantly affect the left atrium. Certain findings indirectly support such a possibility; for example, plasma ANF increases progressively during the genesis of spontaneous hypertension in rats, and this is associated with a relative decrease, compared with age-matched controls, in the concentration of immunoreactive ANF in the left, but not right, atrium (56).

Mechanical distension of the atria or expansion of central blood volume has long been known to provoke diuresis and natriuresis, as well as to decrease plasma renin, aldosterone, and vasopressin (Fig. 9; 47, 56). Early evidence suggested that these responses are mediated in part by stimulation of the cardiopulmonary stretch receptors, leading, via cardiac vagal afferent nerve stimulation, to inhibition of vasopressin release and decreased efferent renal sympathetic nerve traffic. The latter may contribute to the induced natriuresis and inhibition of renin secretion (35, 48). Because ANF infusion has been shown to mimic all responses elicited by atrial distension, it certainly seems possible that increased ANF secretion could contribute as well. There is, in fact, a good correlation between the ANF response to water immersion and the magnitude of the induced natriuresis in normal human subjects (39). A similar correlation does not exist with the associated changes in renin or aldosterone (39), suggesting a dominant effect of neural mechanisms on renin release during acute central blood volume expansion. There is also some evidence that the rise in plasma ANF produced by atrial distension in the denervated heart may, by itself, be insufficient to induce a natriuresis (49). Although the exact role of ANF remains to be defined, available data are consistent with the view of ANF as a hormonal limb to the renal and cardiovascular effects of atrial distension, working in concert with autonomic neural reflexes evoked by activation of atrial stretch receptors.

The potential importance of ANF in the maintenance of chronic sodium balance is less apparent. There are no data to indicate whether the atria are a major monitor of extracellular volume in the long term or whether there are other important regulators of ANF release. Dietary sodium loading increased plasma ANF levels in some preliminary studies (90, 102, 109), but the magnitude of these changes and the degree to which they are sustained is currently debated. Marked expansion of extracellular volume, as occurs in chronic renal parenchymal disease, does appear to be associated with long-term increases in plasma ANF (88). A recent study suggests that ANF may play a role in sustaining renal function in an experimental model of renal failure, since a strong association was found between the rise in plasma ANF and the increases in single-nephron GFR and sodium excretion induced by altered dietary sodium intake (105). Whether a similar situation obtains in the renal adaptation to increased salt intake under normal circumstances remains to be determined.

It seems reasonable to question the physiological relevance of effects that can only be elicited by overtly supraphysiological doses of ANF. There is a pitfall, however, in assuming that the concentrations used in vitro or the plasma levels achieved during infusion must be compared with the levels of endogenous ANF observed in various physiological or pathological states. Even in the case of infusions into intact animals, the situations are not entirely comparable. For example, release of endogenous ANF is provoked by expansion of central blood volume, which simultaneously induces neural reflexes that might well alter target organ responsiveness to the hormone; infusion of the peptide, on the other hand, tends, if anything, to diminish central blood volume. For the moment, therefore, most of the effects that have been described on an impressive array of target organs must be considered potentially significant. Further investigation is needed to assign a relative importance to these actions, both individually and as a whole, in the control of fluid volume and blood pressure.

Many of our colleagues had a major influence on the concepts in this chapter. In particular we thank our associates, Drs. Maria J. F. Camargo, Robert J. Cody, Hollis D. Kleinert, Mark S. Pecker, R. Ernest Sosa, and Massimo Volpe; and our collaborators, Dr. Thomas Maack (Cornell University Medical College), Dr. John Lewicki (California Biotechnology, Inc.), Dr. Murray Epstein (University of Miami School of Medicine), and Dr. Theodore L. Goodfriend (University of Wisconsin). We are also grateful to Linda Stackhouse for her assistance in the preparation of this manuscript.

This work was supported in part by Grant HL-18323-SCR from the National Heart, Lung, and Blood Institute.

REFERENCES

1. ACKERMANN, U., T. G. IRIZAWA, S. MILOJEVIC, AND H. SONNENBERG. Cardiovascular effects of atrial extracts in anesthetized rats. *Can. J. Physiol. Pharmacol.* 62: 819–826, 1984.
2. ALMEIDA, F. A., M. SUZUKI, AND T. MAACK. Atrial natriuretic factor increases hematocrit and decreases plasma volume in nephrectomized rats. *Life Sci.* 39: 1193–1199, 1986.
3. ANAND-SRIVASTAVA, M. B., M. CANTIN, AND J. GENEST. Inhibition of pituitary adenylate cyclase by atrial natriuretic factor. *Life Sci.* 36: 1873–1879, 1985.
4. ANAND-SRIVASTAVA, M. B., D. J. FRANKS, M. CANTIN, AND J. GENEST. Atrial natriuretic factor inhibits adenylate cyclase activity. *Biochem. Biophys. Res. Commun.* 121: 855–862, 1984.
5. ANTUNES-RODRIGUES, J., S. M. MCCANN, L. C. ROGERS, AND W. K. SAMSON. Atrial natriuretic factor inhibits dehydration- and angiotensin II-induced water intake in the conscious, unrestrained rat. *Proc. Natl. Acad. Sci. USA* 82: 8720–8723, 1985.
6. ANTUNES-RODRIGUES, J., S. M. MCCANN, AND W. K. SAMSON. Central administration of atrial natriuretic factor inhibits saline preference in the rat. *Endocrinology* 118: 1726–1728, 1986.

7. ATARASHI, K., P. J. MULROW, AND R. FRANCO-SAENZ. Effect of atrial peptides on aldosterone production. *J. Clin. Invest.* 76: 1807–1811, 1985.

8. ATARASHI, K., P. J. MULROW, R. FRANCO-SAENZ, R. SNAJDAR, AND J. RAPP. Inhibition of aldosterone production by an atrial extract. *Science Wash. DC* 224: 992–994, 1984.

9. ATLAS, S. A. Atrial natriuretic factor: a new hormone of cardiac origin. *Recent Prog. Horm. Res.* 42: 207–249, 1986.

10. ATLAS, S. A., H. D. KLEINERT, M. J. CAMARGO, A. JANUSZEWICZ, J. E. SEALEY, J. H. LARAGH, J. W. SCHILLING, J. A. LEWICKI, L. K. JOHNSON, AND T. MAACK. Purification, sequencing and synthesis of natriuretic and vasoactive rat atrial peptide. *Nature Lond.* 309: 717–720, 1984.

11. ATLAS, S. A., M. VOLPE, R. E. SOSA, J. H. LARAGH, M. J. F. CAMARGO, AND T. MAACK. Effects of atrial natriuretic factor on blood pressure and the renin-angiotensin-aldosterone system. *Federation Proc.* 45: 2115–2121, 1986.

12. BENCOSME, S. A., AND J. M. BERGER. Specific granules in mammalian and non-mammalian vertebrate cardiocytes. In: *Methods of Achievement of Experimental Pathology,* edited by E. Bajusz and G. Jasmin. Basel: Karger, 1971, vol. 5, p. 173.

13. BEX, F., AND A. CORBIN. Atrial natriuretic factor stimulates testosterone production by mouse interstitial cells. *Eur. J. Pharmacol.* 115: 125–126, 1985.

14. BIANCHI, C., J. GUTKOWSKA, G. THIBAULT, R. GARCIA, J. GENEST, AND M. CANTIN. Radioautographic localization of ^{125}I-atrial natriuretic factor (ANF) in rat tissues. *Histochemistry* 82: 441–452, 1985.

15. BORENSTEIN, H. B., W. A. CUPPLES, H. SONNENBERG, AND A. T. VERESS. The effect of a natriuretic atrial extract on renal haemodynamics and urinary excretion in anaesthetized rats. *J. Physiol. Lond.* 334: 133–140, 1983.

16. BURNETT, J. C., JR., J. P. GRANGER, AND T. J. OPGENORTH. Effects of synthetic atrial natriuretic factor on renal function and renin release. *Am. J. Physiol.* 247 (*Renal Fluid Electrolyte Physiol.* 16): F863–F866, 1984.

17. CAMARGO, M. J. F., S. A. ATLAS, AND T. MAACK. Role of increased glomerular filtration rate in atrial natriuretic factor-induced natriuresis in the rat. *Life Sci.* 38: 2397–2404, 1986.

18. CAMARGO, M. J. F., H. D. KLEINERT, S. A. ATLAS, J. E. SEALEY, J. H. LARAGH, AND T. MAACK. Ca-dependent hemodynamic and natriuretic effects of atrial extract in isolated rat kidney. *Am. J. Physiol.* 246 (*Renal Fluid Electrolyte Physiol.* 15): F447–F456, 1984.

19. CAMPBELL, W. B., M. G. CURRIE, AND P. NEEDLEMAN. Inhibition of aldosterone biosynthesis by atriopeptins in rat adrenal cells. *Circ. Res.* 57: 113–118, 1985.

20. CANTIELLO, H. F., AND D. A. AUSIELLO. Atrial natriuretic factor and cGMP inhibit amiloride-sensitive Na^+ transport in the cultured renal epithelial cell line, LLC-PK$_1$. *Biochem. Biophys. Res. Commun.* 134: 852–860, 1986.

21. CANTIN, M., AND J. GENEST. The heart and the atrial natriuretic factor. *Endocr. Rev.* 6: 107–127, 1985.

22. CANTIN, M., J. GUTKOWSKA, G. THIBAULT, R. W. MILNE, S. LEDOUX, S. MINLI, C. CHAPEAU, R. GARCIA, P. HAMET, AND J. GENEST. Immunocytochemical localization of atrial natriuretic factor in the heart and salivary glands. *Histochemistry* 80: 113–127, 1984.

23. CHARTIER, L., E. SCHIFFRIN, AND G. THIBAULT. Effect of atrial natriuretic factor (ANF)-related peptides on aldosterone secretion by adrenal glomerulosa cells: critical role of the intramolecular disulphide bond. *Biochem. Biophys. Res. Commun.* 122: 171–174, 1984.

24. CHARTIER, L., E. L. SCHIFFRIN, G. THIBAULT, AND R. GARCIA. Atrial natriuretic factor inhibits the stimulation of aldosterone secretion by angiotensin II, ACTH and potassium in vitro and angiotensin II-induced steroidogenesis in vivo. *Endocrinology* 115: 2026–2028, 1984.

25. CODY, R. J., S. A. ATLAS, J. H. LARAGH, S. H. KUBO, A. B. COVIT, K. S. RYMAN, A. SHAKNOVICH, K. PONDOLFINO, M. CLARK, M. J. F. CAMARGO, R. M. SCARBOROUGH, AND J. A. LEWICKI. Atrial natriuretic factor in normal subjects and heart failure patients: plasma levels and renal, hormonal and hemodynamic responses to peptide infusion. *J. Clin. Invest.* 78: 1362–1372, 1986.

26. COGAN, M. G. Atrial natriuretic factor can increase renal solute excretion primarily by raising glomerular filtration. *Am. J. Physiol.* 250 (*Renal Fluid Electrolyte Physiol.* 19): F710–F714, 1986.

27. CURRIE, M. G., D. M. GELLER, B. R. COLE, J. G. BOYLAN, W. YUSHENG, S. W. HOLMBERG,

AND P. NEEDLEMAN. Bioactive cardiac substances: potent vasorelaxant activity in mammalian atria. *Science Wash. DC* 221: 71–73, 1983.

28. CURRIE, M. G., D. M. GELLER, B. R. COLE, N. R. SIEGEL, K. F. FOK, S. P. ADAMS, S. R. EUBANKS, G. R. GALLUPPI, AND P. NEEDLEMAN. Purification and sequence analysis of bioactive atrial peptides (atriopeptins). *Science Wash DC* 223: 67–69, 1984.

29. DE BOLD, A. J. Heart atria granularity effects of change in water-electrolyte balance. *Proc. Soc. Exp. Biol. Med.* 161: 508–511, 1979.

30. DE BOLD, A. J. Tissue fractionation studies on the relationship between an atrial natriuretic factor and specific atrial granules. *Can. J. Physiol. Pharmacol.* 60: 324–330, 1982.

31. DE BOLD, A. J. Atrial natriuretic factor: a hormone produced by the heart. *Science Wash. DC* 230: 767–770, 1985.

32. DE BOLD, A. J., H. B. BORENSTEIN, A. T. VERESS, AND H. SONNENBERG. A rapid and potent natriuretic response to intravenous injection of atrial myocardial extract in rats. *Life Sci.* 28: 89–94, 1981.

33. DE LÉAN, A., K. RACZ, J. GUTKOWSKA, T.-T. NGUYEN, M. CANTIN, AND J. GENEST. Specific receptor-mediated inhibition by synthetic atrial natriuretic factor of hormone-stimulated steroidogenesis in cultured bovine adrenal cells. *Endocrinology* 115: 1636–1638, 1984.

34. DETH, R. C., K. WONG, S. FUKOZAWA, R. ROCCO, J. L. SMART, C. J. LYNCH, AND R. AWAD. Inhibition of rat aorta contractile response by natriuresis-inducing extract of rat atrium (abstr.). *Federation Proc.* 41: 983, 1982.

35. DIBONA, G. F. Neural regulation of renal tubular sodium reabsorption and renin secretion. *Federation Proc.* 44: 2816–2822, 1985.

36. DIETZ, J. R. Release of natriuretic factor from rat heart-lung preparation by atrial distension. *Am. J. Physiol.* 247 (*Regulatory Integrative Comp. Physiol.* 16): R1093–R1096, 1984.

37. DILLINGHAM, M. A., AND R. J. ANDERSON. Inhibition of vasopressin action by atrial natriuretic factor. *Science Wash. DC* 231: 1572–1573, 1986.

38. EPSTEIN, M., R. LOUTZENHISER, E. FRIEDLAND, R. M. ACETO, M. J. F. CAMARGO, AND S. A. ATLAS. Increases in circulating atrial natriuretic factor during immerson-induced central hypervolemia in normal humans. *J. Hypertens.* 4, Suppl. 2: S93–S99, 1986.

39. EPSTEIN, M., R. LOUTZENHISER, E. FRIEDLAND, R. M. ACETO, M. J. F. CAMARGO, AND S. A. ATLAS. Relationship of increased plasma ANF and renal sodium handling during immersion-induced central hypervolemia in normal humans. *J. Clin. Invest.* In press.

40. ESPINER, E. A., I. G. CROZIER, M. G. NICHOLLS, R. CUNEO, T. G. YONDLE, AND H. IKRAM. Cardiac secretion of atrial natriuretic peptide. *Lancet* 2: 398–399, 1985.

41. FLYNN, T. G., P. L. DAVIES, B. P. KENNEDY, M. L. DE BOLD, AND A. J. DE BOLD. Alignment of rat cardionatrin sequences with the preprocardionatrin sequence from complementary DNA. *Science Wash. DC* 228: 323–325, 1985.

42. FLYNN, T. G., M. L. DE BOLD, AND A. J. DE BOLD. The amino acid sequence of an atrial peptide with potent diuretic and natriuretic properties. *Biochem. Biophys. Res. Commun.* 117: 859–865, 1983.

43. FRIED, T. A., R. N. McCOY, R. W. OSGOOD, H. J. REINECK, AND J. H. STEIN. The effect of atrial natriuretic peptide on glomerular hemodynamics (abstr.). *Clin. Res.* 33: 584a, 1985.

44. GARCIA, R., M. CANTIN, G. THIBAULT, H. ONG, AND J. GENEST. Relationship of specific granules to the natriuretic and diuretic activity of rat atria. *Experientia Basel* 38: 1071–1073, 1982.

45. GARCIA, R., G. THIBAULT, J. GUTKOWSKA, M. CANTIN, AND J. GENEST. Changes of regional blood flow induced by atrial natriuretic factor (ANF) in conscious rats. *Life Sci.* 36: 1687–1692, 1985.

46. GARCIA, R., G. THIBAULT, J. GUTKOWSKA, P. HAMET, M. CANTIN, AND J. GENEST. Effect of chronic infusion of synthetic atrial natriuretic factor (ANF 8-33) in conscious two-kidney, one-clip hypertensive rats. *Proc. Soc. Exp. Biol. Med.* 178: 155–159, 1985.

47. GAUER, O. H., J. P. HENRY, AND H. O. SIEKER. Cardiac receptors and fluid volume control. *Prog. Cardiovasc. Dis.* 4: 1–26, 1961.

48. GOETZ, K. L., G. C. BOND, AND D. D. BLOXHAM. Atrial receptors and renal function. *Physiol. Rev.* 55: 157–205, 1975.

49. GOETZ, K. L., B. C. WANG, P. G. GEER, R. J. LEADLEY, JR., AND H. W. REINHARDT. Atrial stretch increases sodium excretion independently of release of atrial peptides. *Am. J. Physiol.* 250 (*Regulatory Integrative Comp. Physiol.* 19): R946–R950, 1986.

50. GOODFRIEND, T. L., M. ELLIOTT, AND S. A. ATLAS. Actions of synthetic atrial natriuretic factor on bovine adrenal glomerulosa. *Life Sci.* 35: 1675–1682, 1984.

51. GRAMMER, R. T., H. FUKUMI, T. INAGAMI, AND K. S. MISONO. Rat atrial natriuretic factor.

Purification and vasorelaxant activity. *Biochem. Biophys. Res. Commun.* 116: 696–703, 1983.

52. HAMET P., J. TREMBLAY, S. C. PANG, R. GARCIA, G. THIBAULT, J. GUTKOWSKA, M. CANTIN, AND J. GENEST. Effect of native and synthetic atrial natriuretic factor on cyclic GMP. *Biochem. Biophys. Res. Commun.* 123: 515–527, 1984.

53. HEISLER, S., J. SIMAND, E. ASSAYAG, Y. MEHRI, AND F. LABRIE. Atrial natriuretic factor does not affect basal, forskolin- and CRF-stimulated adenylate cyclase activity, cAMP formation or ACTH secretion but does stimulate cGMP synthesis in anterior pituitary. *Mol. Cell Endocrinol.* 44: 125–131, 1986.

54. HUANG, C. L., J. LEWICKI, L. K. JOHNSON, AND M. G. COGAN. Renal mechanism of action of rat atrial natriuretic factor. *J. Clin. Invest.* 75: 769–773, 1985.

55. ICHIKAWA, I., B. R. DUNN, J. L. TRAY, T. MAACK, AND B. M. BRENNER. Influence of atrial natriuretic peptide on glomerular microcirculation in vivo (abstr.). *Clin. Res.* 33: 487A, 1985.

56. IMADA, T., R. TAKAYANAGI, AND T. INAGAMI. Changes in the content of atrial natriuretic factor with the progression of hypertension in spontaneously hypertensive rats. *Biochem. Biophys. Res. Commun.* 133: 759–765, 1985.

57. ISHIHARA, T., K. AISAKA, K. HATTORI, S. HAMASAKI, M. MORITA, T. NOGUCHI, K. KANGAWA, AND H. MATSUO. Vasodilatory and diuretic actions of α-human atrial natriuretic polypeptide (α-hANP). *Life Sci.* 36: 1205–1215, 1985.

58. JACOBOWITZ, D. M., G. SKOFITSCH, H. R. KEISER, R. L. ESKAY, AND N. ZAMIR. Evidence for the existence of atrial natriuretic factor-containing neurons in the rat brain. *Neuroendocrinology* 40: 92–94, 1985.

59. JAMIESON, J. D., AND G. E. PALADE. Specific granules in atrial muscle cells. *J. Cell Biol.* 23: 151–172, 1964.

60. JANUSZEWICZ, P., J. GUTKOWSKA, A. DE LÉAN, G. THIBAULT, R. GARCIA, J. GENEST, AND M. CANTIN. Synthetic atrial natriuretic factor induces release (possibly receptor-mediated) of vasopressin from rat posterior pituitary. *Proc. Soc. Exp. Biol. Med.* 178: 321–325, 1985.

61. KANGAWA, K., AND H. MATSUO. Purification and complete amino acid sequence of alpha-human atrial natriuretic polypeptide (α-hANP). *Biochem. Biophys. Res. Commun.* 118: 131–139, 1984.

62. KANGAWA, K., Y. TAWARAGI, S. OIKAWA, A. MIZUNO, Y. SAKURAGAWA, H. NAKAZATO, A. FUKUDA, N. MINAMINO, AND H. MATSUO. Identification of rat gamma-atrial natriuretic polypeptide and characterization of the cDNA encoding its precursor. *Nature Lond.* 312: 152–155, 1984.

63. KISCH, B. Electron microscopy of the atrium of the heart. I. Guinea pig. *Exp. Med. Surg.* 114: 99–112, 1956.

64. KLEINERT, H. D., T. MAACK, S. A. ATLAS, A. JANUSZEWICZ, J. E. SEALEY, AND J. H. LARAGH. Atrial natriuretic factor inhibits angiotensin-, norepinephrine-, and potassium-induced vascular contractility. *Hypertension Dallas* 6, Suppl. I: I143–I147, 1984.

65. KLEINERT, H. D., M. VOLPE, G. ODELL, D. MARION, S. A. ATLAS, M. J. F. CAMARGO, J. H. LARAGH, AND T. MAACK. Cardiovascular effects of synthetic atrial natriuretic factor in anesthetized and conscious dogs. *Hypertension Dallas* 8: 312–316, 1986.

66. KOBRIN, I., M. B. KARDON, N. C. TRIPPODO, B. L. PEGRAM, AND E. D. FROLICH. Renal response to acute volume overload in conscious rats with atrial appendectomy. *J. Hypertens.* 3: 145–148, 1985.

67. KUDO, T., AND A. BAIRD. Inhibition of aldosterone production in the adrenal glomerulosa by atrial natriuretic factor. *Nature Lond.* 312: 756–757, 1984.

68. LANG, R. E., H. THÖLKEN, D. GANTEN, F. C. LUFT, H. RUSKOAHO, AND T. H. UNGER. Atrial natriuretic factor—a circulating hormone, stimulated by volume loading. *Nature Lond.* 314: 264–266, 1985.

69. LAPPE, R. W., J. F. M. SMITS, J. A. TODT, J. J. M. DEBETS, AND R. L. WENDT. Failure of atriopeptin II to cause arterial vasodilation in the conscious rat. *Circ. Res.* 56: 606–612, 1985.

70. LEDSOME, J. R., N. WILSON, C. A. COURNEYA, AND A. J. RANKIN. Release of atrial natriuretic peptide by atrial distension. *Can. J. Physiol. Pharmacol.* 63: 739–742, 1985.

71. MAACK, T., M. J. F. CAMARGO, H. D. KLEINERT, J. H. LARAGH, AND S. A. ATLAS. Atrial natriuretic factor: structure and functional properties. *Kidney Int.* 27: 607–615, 1985.

72. MAACK, T., D. N. MARION, M. J. F. CAMARGO, H. D. KLEINERT, J. H. LARAGH, E. D. VAUGHAN, JR., AND S. A. ATLAS. Effects of auriculin (atrial natriuretic factor) on blood

pressure, renal function, and the renin-aldosterone system in dogs. *Am. J. Med.* 77: 1069–1075, 1984.

73. MAKI, M., R. TAKAYANAGI, K. S. MISONA, K. N. PANDEY, C. TIBBETTS, AND T. INAGAMI. Structure of rat atrial natriuretic factor precursor deduced from cDNA sequence. *Nature Lond.* 309: 722–724, 1984.

74. MANNING, P. T., D. SCHWARTZ, N. C. KATSUBE, S. W. HOLMBERG, AND P. NEEDLEMAN. Vasopressin-stimulated release of atriopeptin: endocrine antagonists in fluid homeostasis. *Science Wash. DC* 229: 395–397, 1985.

75. MARIE, J. P., H. GUILLEMOT, AND P. Y. HATT. Le degré de granulation des cardiocytes auriculaires. Etude planimétrique au cours de différents apports d'eau et du sodium chez le rat. *Pathol. Biol.* 24: 549–554, 1976.

76. MISONO, K. S., R. T. GRAMMER, H. FUKUMI, AND T. INAGAMI. Rat atrial natriuretic factor: isolation, structure and biological activities of four major peptides. *Biochem. Biophys. Res. Commun.* 123: 444–451, 1984.

77. NAKAMURA, M., G. KATSUURA, K. NAKAO, AND H. IMURA. Antidipsogenic action of α-human atrial natriuretic polypeptide administered intracerebroventricularly in rats. *Neurosci. Lett.* 58: 1–6, 1985.

78. NARUSE, M., K. OBANA, K. NARUSE, N. SUGINO, H. DEMURA, K. SHIZUME, AND T. INAGAMI. Antisera to atrial natriuretic factor reduces urinary sodium excretion and increases plasma renin activity in rats. *Biochem. Biophys. Res. Commun.* 132: 954–960, 1985.

79. NEEDLEMAN, P., S. P. ADAMS, B. R. COLE, M. G. CURRIE, D. M. GELLER, M. L. MICHENER, C. B. SAPER, D. SCHWARTZ, AND D. G. STANDAERT. Atriopeptins as cardiac hormones. *Hypertension Dallas* 7: 469–482, 1985.

80. OBANA, K., M. NARUSE, T. INAGAMI, A. B. BROWN, K. NARUSE, F. KURIMENTO, H. SAKURAI, H. DEMURA, AND K. SHIZUME. Atrial natriuretic factor inhibits vasopressin secretion from rat posterior pituitary. *Biochem. Biophys. Res. Commun.* 132: 1088–1094, 1985.

81. OBANA, K., M. NARUSE, K. NARUSE, H. SAKURAI, H. DEMURA, T. INAGAMI, AND K. SHIZUME. Synthetic rat atrial natriuretic factor inhibits in vitro and in vivo renin secretion in rats. *Endocrinology* 117: 1282–1284, 1985.

82. OIKAWA, S., M. IMAI, A. UENO, S. TANAKA, T. NOGUCHI, H. NAKAZATO, K. KANGAWA, A. FUKUDA, AND H. MATSUO. Cloning and sequence analysis of cDNA encoding a precursor for human atrial natriuretic polypeptide. *Nature Lond.* 309: 724–726, 1984.

83. OPGENORTH, T. J., J. C. BURNETT, JR., J. P. GRANGER, AND T. A. SCRIVEN. Effects of atrial natriuretic peptide on renin secretion in nonfiltering kidney. *Am. J. Physiol.* 250 (*Renal Fluid Electrolyte Physiol.* 19): F798–F801, 1986.

84. OSHIMA, T., M. G. CURRIE, D. M. GELLER, AND P. NEEDLEMAN. An atrial peptide is a potent renal vasodilator substance. *Circ. Res.* 54: 612–616, 1984.

85. PANDEY, K. N., W. J. KOVACS, AND T. INAGAMI. The inhibition of progesterone secretion and the regulation of cyclic nucleotides by atrial natriuretic factor in gonadotropin responsive murine Leydig tumor cells. *Biochem. Biophys. Res. Commun.* 133: 800–806, 1985.

86. PEGRAM, B. L., M. B. KARDON, N. C. TRIPPODO, F. E. COLE, AND A. A. MACPHEE. Atrial extract: hemodynamics in Wistar-Kyoto and spontaneously hypertensive rats. *Am. J. Physiol.* 249 (*Heart Circ. Physiol.* 18): H265–H271, 1985.

87. QUIRION, R., M. DALPÉ, A. DE LÉAN, J. GUTKOWSKA, M. CANTIN, AND J. GENEST. Atrial natriuretic factor (ANF) binding sites in brain and related structures. *Peptides* 5: 1167–1172, 1984.

88. RASCHER, W., T. TULASSAY, AND R. E. LANG. Atrial natriuretic peptide in plasma of volume overloaded children with chronic renal failure. *Lancet* 2: 303–305, 1985.

89. RICHARDS, A. M., H. IKRAM, T. G. YONDLE, M. G. NICHOLLS, M. W. I. WEBSTER, AND E. A. ESPINER. Renal, hemodynamic and hormonal effects of human alpha atrial natriuretic peptide in healthy volunteers. *Lancet* 1: 545–549, 1985.

90. SAGNELLA, G. A., N. D. MARKANDU, A. C. SHORE, AND G. A. MACGREGOR. Effects of changes in dietary sodium intake and saline infusion on immunoreactive atrial natriuretic peptide in human plasma. *Lancet* 2: 1208–1210, 1985.

91. SAMSON, W. K. Atrial natriuretic factor inhibits dehydration and hemorrhage-induced vasopressin release. *Neuroendocrinology* 40: 277–279, 1985.

92. SAMSON, W. K. Dehydration-induced alterations in rat brain vasopressin and atrial natriuretic factor immunoreactivity. *Endocrinology* 117: 1279–1281, 1985.

93. SAMSON, W. K., AND R. L. ESKAY. Endocrine and neuroendocrine actions of cardiac peptides.

In: *Neural and Endocrine Peptides and Receptors*, edited by T. W. Moody. New York: Plenum, in press.

94. SAMSON, W. K., AND J. C. VANATTA. Atrial natriuretic factor inhibits vasotocin-induced water reabsorption in the toad urinary bladder. *Proc. Soc. Exp. Biol. Med.* 181: 169–172, 1986.

95. SAPER, C. B., D. G. STANDAERT, M. G. CURRIE, D. SCHWARTZ, D. M. GELLER, AND P. NEEDLEMAN. Atriopeptin-immunoreactive neurons in the brain: presence in cardiovascular regulatory areas. *Science Wash. DC* 227: 1047–1049, 1985.

96. SASAKI, A., O. KIDA, K. KANGAWA, H. MATSUO, AND K. TANAKA. Hemodynamic effects of α-human natriuretic polypeptide (α-hANP) in rats. *Eur. J. Pharmacol.* 109: 405–407, 1985.

97. SCHENCK, D. B., L. K. JOHNSON, K. SCHWARTZ, H. SISTA, R. M. SCARBOROUGH, AND J. A. LEWICKI. *Biochem. Biophys. Res. Commun.* 127: 433–442, 1985.

98. SCHWARTZ, D., D. M. GELLER, P. T. MANNING, N. R. SIEGEL, K. F. FOK, C. E. SMITH, AND P. NEEDLEMAN. Ser-Leu-Arg-Arg-atriopeptin III: the major circulating form of atrial peptide. *Science Wash. DC* 229: 397–400, 1985.

99. SEIDAH, N. G., C. LAZURE, M. CHRÉTIEN, G. THIBAULT, R. GARCIA, M. CANTIN, J. GENEST, R. F. NUTT, S. F. BRADY, T. A. LYLE, W. J. PALAVEDA, C. D. COLTON, T. M. CICCARONE, AND D. F. VEBER. Amino acid sequence of homologous rat atrial peptides: natriuretic activity of native and synthetic forms. *Proc. Natl. Acad. Sci. USA* 81: 2640–2644, 1984.

100. SEIDMAN, C. E., A. D. DUBY, E. CHOI, R. M. GRAHAM, E. HABER, C. HOMCY, J. A. SMITH, AND J. G. SEIDMAN. The structure of rat preproatrial natriuretic factor as defined by a complementary DNA clone. *Science Wash. DC* 225: 324–326, 1984.

101. SEYMOUR, A. A., E. A. MARSH, E. K. MAZACK, I. I. STABILITO, AND E. H. BLAINE. Synthetic atrial natriuretic factor in conscious normotensive and hypertensive rats. *Hypertension Dallas* 7, Suppl. I: I35–I42, 1985.

102. SHENKER, Y., R. S. SIDER, E. A. OSTAFIN, AND R. J. GREKIN. Plasma levels of immunoreactive atrial natriuretic factor in healthy subjects and in patients with edema. *J. Clin. Invest.* 76: 1684–1698, 1985.

103. SHIBASAKI, T., M. NARUSE, N. YAMAUCHI, A. MASUDA, T. IMAKI, K. NARUSE, H. DEMURA, N. LING, T. INAGAMI, AND K. SHIZUME. Rat atrial natriuretic factor suppresses proopiomelanocortin-derived peptides secretion from both anterior and intermediate lobe cells and growth hormone release from anterior lobe cells of rat pituitary in vitro. *Biochem. Biophys. Res. Commun.* 135: 1035–1041, 1986.

104. SKOFITSCH, G., D. M. JACOBOWITZ, R. L. ESKAY, AND N. ZAMIR. Distribution of atrial natriuretic factor-like immunoreactive neurons in brain. *Neuroscience* 16: 917–948, 1985.

105. SMITH, S., S. ANDERSON, B. J. BALLERMANN, AND B. M. BRENNER. Role of atrial natriuretic peptide in adaptation of sodium excretion with reduced renal mass. *J. Clin. Invest.* 77: 1395–1398, 1986.

106. SNAJDAR, R. M., AND J. P. RAPP. Atrial natriuretic factor in Dahl rats. Atrial content and renal and aortic responses. *Hypertension Dallas* 7: 775–782, 1985.

107. SOSA, R. E., M. VOLPE, D. N. MARION, S. A. ATLAS, J. H. LARAGH, E. D. VAUGHAN, JR., AND T. MAACK. Relationship between renal hemodynamic and natriuretic effects of atrial natriuretic factor. *Am. J. Physiol.* 250 (*Renal Fluid Electrolyte Physiol.* 19): F520–F524, 1986.

108. SOSA, R. E., M. VOLPE, D. N. MARION, N. GLORIOSO, J. H. LARAGH, E. D. VAUGHAN, JR., T. MAACK, AND S. A. ATLAS. Effect of atrial natriuretic factor on renin secretion, plasma renin and aldosterone in dogs with acute unilateral renal artery constriction. *J. Hypertens.* 3, Suppl. 3: S299–S302, 1985.

109. TANAKA, I., K. S. MISONO, AND T. INAGAMI. Atrial natriuretic factor in rat hypothalamus, atria and plasma: determination by specific radioimmunoassay. *Biochem. Biophys. Res. Commun.* 124: 663–668, 1984.

110. THIBAULT, G., C. LAZURE, E. L. SCHIFFRIN, J. GUTKOWSKA, L. CHARTIER, R. GARCIA, N. G. SEIDAH, M. CHRÉTIEN, J. GENEST, AND M. CANTIN. Identification of a biologically active circulating form of rat atrial natriuretic factor. *Biochem. Biophys. Res. Commun.* 130: 981–986, 1985.

111. TIKKANEN, I., R. FYHRQUIST, K. METSÄRINNE, AND R. LEIDENIUS. Plasma atrial natriuretic peptide in cardiac disease and during infusion in healthy volunteers. *Lancet* 2: 66–69, 1985.

112. TREMBLAY, J., R. GERZER, P. VINAY, S. C. PANG, R. BÉLIVEAU, AND P. HAMET. The

increase of cGMP by atrial natriuretic factor correlates with the distribution of particulate guanylate cyclase. *FEBS Lett.* 181: 17–22, 1985.

113. VERESS, A. T., AND H. SONNENBERG. Right atrial appendectomy reduces the renal response to acute hypervolemia in the rat. *Am. J. Physiol.* 247: (*Regulatory Integrative Comp. Physiol.* 16): R610–R613, 1984.

114. VOLPE, M., G. ODELL, H. D. KLEINERT, M. J. F. CAMARGO, J. H. LARAGH, J. A. LEWICKI, T. MAACK, E. D. VAUGHAN, JR., AND S. A. ATLAS. Antihypertensive and aldosterone lowering effects of synthetic atrial natriuretic factor in renin dependent renovascular hypertension. *J. Hypertens.* 2, Suppl. 3: 313–315, 1984.

115. VOLPE, M., G. ODELL, H. D. KLEINERT, F. MULLER, M. J. F. CAMARGO, J. H. LARAGH, T. MAACK, E. D. VAUGHAN, JR., AND S. A. ATLAS. Effect of atrial natriuretic factor on blood pressure, renin and aldosterone in Goldblatt hypertension. *Hypertension Dallas* 7, Suppl. I: I43–I48, 1985.

116. VOLPE, M., R. E. SOSA, F. B. MÜLLER, M. J. F. CAMARGO, N. GLORIOSO, J. H. LARAGH, T. MAACK, AND S. A. ATLAS. Differing hemodynamic responses to atrial natriuretic factor in two models of hypertension. *Am. J. Physiol.* 250 (*Heart Circ. Physiol.* 19): H871–H878, 1986.

117. WALDMAN, S. A., R. M. RAPOPORT, AND F. MURAD. Atrial natriuretic factor selectively activates particulate guanylate cyclase and elevates cyclic GMP in rat tissues. *J. Biol. Chem.* 259: 14332–14334, 1984.

118. WEIDMANN, P., L. HASLER, M. P. GNÄDINGER, R. E. LANG, D. E. UEHLINGER, S. SHAW, W. RASCHER, AND F. C. REUBI. Blood levels and renal effects of atrial natriuretic peptide in normal man. *J. Clin. Invest.* 77: 734–742, 1986.

119. WINQUIST, R. J., E. P. FAISON, AND R. F. NUTT. Vasodilator profile of synthetic atrial natriuretic factor. *Eur. J. Pharmacol.* 102: 169–173, 1984.

120. WINQUIST, R. J., E. P. FAISON, S. A. WALDMAN, K. SCHWARTZ, F. MURAD, AND R. M. RAPOPORT. Atrial natriuretic factor elicits an endothelium-independent relaxation and activates particulate guanylate cyclase in vascular smooth muscle. *Proc. Natl. Acad. Sci. USA* 81: 7661–7664, 1984.

121. YAMAJI, T., M. ISHIBASHI, H. NAKAOKA, K. IMATAKA, M. AMANO, AND J. FUJII. Possible role for atrial natriuretic peptide in polyuria associated with paroxysmal atrial arrhythmias (letter to the editor). *Lancet* 1: 1211, 1985.

122. YAMAJI, T., M. ISHIBASHI, AND F. TAKAKU. Atrial natriuretic factor in human blood. *J. Clin. Invest.* 76: 1705–1709, 1985.

123. YAMANAKA, M., B. GREENBERG, L. JOHNSON, J. SEILHAMER, M. BREWER, T. FRIEDMANN, J. MILLER, S. ATLAS, J. LARAGH, J. LEWICKI, AND J. FIDDES. Cloning and sequence analysis of cDNA for the rat atrial natriuretic factor precursor. *Nature Lond.* 309: 719–722, 1984.

Structure-Activity Relationships
of Atrial Natriuretic Peptides

GAÉTAN THIBAULT, RAUL GARCIA, ERNESTO L. SCHIFFRIN,
ANDRÉ DE LÉAN, PETER W. SCHILLER, JOLANTA GUTKOWSKA,
JACQUES GENEST, AND MARC CANTIN

Clinical Research Institute of Montreal, Montreal, Canada

Biological Assays
Binding Assays

SINCE THE INITIAL OBSERVATION of de Bold and co-workers (1), the atrial natriuretic factor (ANF) has been developed into a new hormonal system that appears to play an important role in salt and water homeostasis and blood pressure. The primary structure of this factor is now well characterized. Its precursor is composed of 126 amino acids and contains a disulfide bridge between Cys105 and Cys121. The 28 amino acids at the COOH-terminal sequence represent the circulating form. In the rat, rabbit, and mouse, ANF peptides contain isoleucine in position 110, which is substituted by methionine in the human, dog, and bovine sequences.

Initially, once the structure of ANF was elucidated, many peptides varying in length from 21 to 33 amino acids were sequenced. Physiological studies were undertaken with some of these peptides without precise knowledge of their biological potency. We have therefore begun an extensive study of the influence of the length of various ANF peptides on different physiological parameters. From ANF (Arg101-Tyr126) we produced truncated peptides either at the COOH-terminal by using carboxypeptidases or at the NH_2-terminal by Edman degradation (18). The ANF (Gly96-Tyr126) and ANF (Glu54-Tyr126) were obtained by purification (15, 17). The ANF (Ser99-Tyr126), human ANF (Ser99-Tyr126), and the atriopeptins were obtained either from Peninsula Laboratories (Belmont, CA) or from Institut Armand-Frappier (Laval, Quebec, Canada). The ANF (Phe106-Tyr126) was produced by solid-phase synthesis (13). These various peptides have been systematically assayed on a variety of biological and binding assays.

BIOLOGICAL ASSAYS

The first biological assay used to screen ANF in atrial extracts or in fractions during purification procedures was the natriuretic assay. The material was injected into anesthetized rats and the increase of diuresis and natriuresis recorded. The natriuretic assay is not very sensitive: at least 100 pmol of peptide were necessary to significantly increase sodium urinary excretion (15). A plateau was obtained with doses >2,000 pmol. Analysis of the potency of various ANF peptides on natriuresis is shown in Table 1. All the NH$_2$-terminal extended or truncated peptides demonstrated a comparable degree of natriuretic activity. The variability of the natriuretic assay is such that a twofold difference was not significant. Only deletions of the residues 122–126 at the COOH-terminal, as in ANF (Arg101-Cys121), resulted in reduction of the natriuretic activity. In the dog, as Needleman et al. (10) reported, natriuresis was not affected by deletion of residues 99–102. Further removal of the NH$_2$-terminal residues or amino acids 126–124 at the COOH-terminal reduces sodium excretion by a factor of 10. In fact, in vivo assays, such as the natriuresis assay, are not good systems to assess peptide potency, since either proteolysis in the circulation or the physiological state of each animal may affect the response.

The ANF is a potent relaxant of contracted vascular and nonvascular smooth muscle. Relaxation of precontracted chick rectum proved to be another useful biological assay to screen ANF activity (5). The sensitivity of that assay was at least 10 times greater than the natriuretic one, since as little as 10 pmol of ANF can be detected. The potency of the peptides evaluated by this assay is shown in Table 1. The ANF (Ser99-Tyr126), ANF (Arg101-Tyr126), and ANF (Cys105-Tyr126) demonstrated the highest activity. Interestingly, deletion of Arg101 and Arg102 decreased the activity, but further removal of Ser103 and Ser104 seems to restore it completely. Here again, deletion of Phe-Arg-Tyr at the COOH-terminal was critical.

Relaxation of norepinephrine-contracted vascular tissue, such as the

TABLE 1. *Relative biological potency of ANF-related peptides*

ANF Peptides	Sodium Excretion	Relaxation		Aldosterone Inhibition	
		Chick rectum	Rabbit aorta	Bovine adrenal cells	Rat adrenal cells
54–126	44		0.2	63	
96–126	57		32	253	
99–126	51	122	127	100	100
101–126	100	100	100	100	100
102–126	133	36	100	100	
103–126	95	15	10	100	20
104–126	86	76	8	32	
105–126	143	162	32	32	
101–125	116	74	4	1,000	150
101–124	75		0.4		
101–123	21	43	0.2	3	5
101–121	3	21	0.1	1	
103–125	42	9	0.6	63	20
103–123	22	5	0.3	0.3	5
106–125		0.5	0.004	0.1	
Met[110] (99–126)					30

All potencies were calculated by comparison with ANF (Arg101-Tyr126).

rabbit aorta, gave essentially the same results as the relaxation of intestinal smooth muscle (4). These results were further exemplified by studying the vasodilatation effects of ANF. On isolated rat or dog kidney, the longer peptides, such as ANF (Ser99-Tyr126), were the most effective in increasing renal blood flow, which was secondary to a decrease in renal vascular resistance (9, 20). However, most of the peptides produced an equivalent fall of blood pressure in intact animals (21), suggesting that, as for the natriuretic assay, in vivo experiments may not be adequate to evaluate accurately the potency of such peptides.

When cells of adrenal zona glomerulosa were incubated in the presence of ANF, an inhibition of aldosterone secretion was observed. This inhibition was seen on the basal as well as on the stimulated secretion. Fifty percent of inhibition was observed with an ANF concentration of 50–200 pM (2, 11). Deletion of the last three COOH-terminal residues drastically reduced the inhibitory effects of ANF on aldosterone secretion. However, the removal of the two last NH_2-terminal residues preceding the Cys105 affected only slightly that activity (Table 1).

The biological response to ANF appears to be partly mediated by activation of the particulate guanylate cyclase followed by enhanced production of cGMP (6, 22). Whether cGMP is the prime messenger of the biological action is not known. Partial data indicate that a lower biological response to ANF peptides is accompanied by a lower efficiency of these peptides to stimulate the production of cGMP (7).

BINDING ASSAYS

The observation of the various physiological effects of ANF was followed by the finding that binding sites for ANF were located in the same target tissues. Binding sites for ANF have been reported in many tissues. In Table 2 the relative potency of the dissociation constant of related ANFs on some tissue preparations is presented. Binding was examined on membrane preparations of rat and bovine adrenal zona glomerulosa, rat mesenteric arteries, and human platelets (2, 11, 12). In general the truncated ANFs demonstrated the same potency on all these tissue preparations. The potency was slightly affected by the removal of Arg101, but further deletion of residues at the NH_2-terminal decreased it. Deletion of Phe-Arg at the COOH-terminal side decreased binding.

Analysis of the data in Tables 1 and 2 indicates a fairly good correlation between the binding affinities to the truncated ANFs and the levels of the biological responses, indicating, therefore, that the binding sites for ANF correspond to true receptors. These receptors are associated in all cases with biological response, which may be production of cGMP, sodium excretion, smooth muscle relaxation, or steroidogenesis inhibition. The significance of platelet-binding sites remains to be demonstrated.

The following general comments can be drawn from the previous results.

TABLE 2. *Relative binding potency of ANF-related peptides*

ANF Peptides	Binding to			
	Rat adrenal cells	Rat mesenteric arteries	Bovine adrenal cells	Human platelets
54–126	107	148	32	
96–126	122	150	100	
99–126	100	200	158	
101–126	100	100	100	100
102–126	24	20	100	
103–126	20	20	10	41
104–126	13	18	13	
105–126	11	29	8	
101–125	190	150	250	
101–124	37	39	6	
101–123	35	40	0.3	
101–121	31	26	0.08	
103–125	6	15	8	18
103–123	11	5	0.02	7
106–125			0.004	
Met[110] (99–126)	81	77	63	90

All values were calculated by comparison with ANF (Arg101-Tyr126).

The maximal potency was obtained with ANF (Arg101-Tyr126) and ANF (Ser99-Tyr126) (3). This last peptide is also the circulating form of ANF (14, 19). Addition of amino acids at the NH_2-terminal, like ANF (Glu54-Tyr126), affected only slightly the biological and the binding potency. The precursor of ANF is approximately five times less potent (8). These data seem also to indicate that, on the assays used, there is no tissue or species specificity. Truncated peptides demonstrated comparable potency on rat, human, rabbit, bovine, and chicken tissues. This is further exemplified with human ANF, which gives identical responses on rat, bovine, and human tissue.

Human and rat ANF show similar potency, suggesting that the methionine residue in position 110 may not be involved in the binding of ANF to its receptor. This was further confirmed by Seymour et al. (16), who observed comparable degrees of vasodilatation, sodium excretion, and renin inhibition in the conscious dog.

Studies done with ANF (Phe106-Tyr126) suggest the importance of the disulfide bridge in the conformational structure of ANF and therefore for its binding. The linear peptide, which is ~1,000 times less potent than ANF (Arg101-Tyr126), had very low biological activity. However, it is still active at concentrations in the micromolar range, indicating that the loop conformation is not an absolute requirement for biological activity.

Removal of NH_2-terminal residues from Arg101 to Cys105 reduces progressively the potency by a factor of 10. These amino acids, in particular Arg102 and Ser103, are probably important in the stabilization of ANF binding to its receptors. On the other hand, deletion of COOH-terminal residues, with the exception of Tyr126, decreased by a factor of 100 the binding and consequently the biological responses.

Interestingly, simultaneous deletion of amino acids at both ends, as in atriopeptin I [ANF (Ser103-Ser123)], caused additive deleterious effects. The ANF (Ser103-Arg125) elicited a response similar to that of ANF (Ser103-Tyr126), since the Tyr126 did not seem necessary for the activity.

In conclusion, the amino acids flanking the disulfide bridge, in particular those at the COOH-terminal, as well as the disulfide bridge, are necessary to express the full biological activity. The circulating forms ANF (Ser99-Tyr126) and ANF (Arg101-Tyr126) are equipotent and elicit the maximal physiological response.

REFERENCES

1. DE BOLD, A. J., H. B. BORENSTEIN, A. T. VERESS, AND H. SONNENBERG. A rapid and potent natriuretic response to intravenous injection of atrial myocardial extract in rats. *Life Sci.* 28: 89–94, 1981.
2. DE LÉAN, A., G. THIBAULT, N. G. SEIDAH, C. LAZURE, J. GUTKOWSKA, M. CHRÉTIEN, J. GENEST, AND M. CANTIN. Structure-activity relationships of atrial natriuretic factor (ANF). III. Correlation of receptor affinity with relative potency on aldosterone production in zona glomerulosa cells. *Biochem. Biophys. Res. Commun.* 132: 360–367, 1985.
3. GARCIA, R., M. CANTIN, A. DE LÉAN, J. GENEST, J. GODIN, J. GUTKOWSKA, E. L. SCHIFFRIN, AND G. THIBAULT. Comparative biological activities of ANF (Arg101-Tyr126) and the synthetic form of circulating ANF (Ser99-Tyr126). *Biochem. Biophys. Res. Commun.* 135: 987–993, 1986.
4. GARCIA, R., G. THIBAULT, N. G. SEIDAH, C. LAZURE, M. CANTIN, J. GENEST, AND M. CHRÉTIEN. Structure-activity relationships of atrial natriuretic factor (ANF). II. Effect of chain-length modifications on vascular reactivity. *Biochem. Biophys. Res. Commun.* 126: 178–184, 1985.
5. GELLER, D. M., M. G. CURRIE, K. WAKITANI, B. R. COLE, S. P. ADAMS, K. F. FOK, N. R. SIEGEL, S. R. EUBANKS, G. R. GALLUPI, AND P. NEEDLEMAN. Atriopeptins: a family of potent biologically active peptides derived from mammalian atria. *Biochem. Biophys. Res. Commun.* 120: 333–338, 1984.
6. HAMET, P., J. TREMBLAY, S. C. PANG, R. GARCIA, G. THIBAULT, J. GUTKOWSKA, M. CANTIN, AND J. GENEST. Effect of native and synthetic atrial natriuretic factor on cyclic GMP. *Biochem. Biophys. Res. Commun.* 123: 515–527, 1984.
7. HAMET, P., J. TREMBLAY, S. C. PANG, R. SKUKERSKA, E. L. SCHIFFRIN, R. GARCIA, M. CANTIN, J. GENEST, R. PALMOUR, F. R. ERVIN, S. MARTIN, AND R. GOLDWATER. Cyclic GMP as mediator and biological marker of atrial natriuretic factor. *J. Hypertens.* 4, Suppl. 2: 549–556, 1986.
8. KANGAWA, K., A. FUKUDA, AND H. MATSUO. Structural identification of β- and α-human atrial natriuretic polypeptides. *Nature Lond.* 313: 397–400, 1985.
9. KATSUBE, N., K. WAKITANI, K. F. FOK, F. S. TJOENG, M. E. ZUPEC, S. R. EUBANKS, S. P. ADAMS, AND P. NEEDLEMAN. Differential structure-activity relationships of atrial peptides as natriuretics and renal vasodilators in the dog. *Biochem. Biophys. Res. Commun.* 128: 325–330, 1985.
10. NEEDLEMAN, P., S. P. ADAMS, B. R. COLE, M. G. CURRIE, D. M. GELLER, M. L. MICHENER, C. B. SAPER, D. SCHWARTZ, AND D. G. STANDAERT. Atriopeptins as cardiac hormones. *Hypertension Dallas* 7: 469–482, 1985.
11. SCHIFFRIN, E. L., L. CHARTIER, G. THIBAULT, J. ST-LOUIS, M. CANTIN, AND J. GENEST. Vascular and adrenal receptors for atrial natriuretic factor in the rat. *Circ. Res.* 56: 801–807, 1985.
12. SCHIFFRIN, E. L., M. DESLONGCHAMPS, AND G. THIBAULT. Platelet binding sites for atrial natriuretic factor in humans. Characterization and effects of sodium intake. *Hypertension Dallas* 8, Suppl. II: II6–II10, 1986.
13. SCHILLER, P. W., L. MAZIAK, T. M. D. NGUYEN, J. GODIN, R. GARCIA, A. DE LÉAN, AND M. CANTIN. Synthesis and biological activity of a linear fragment of the atrial natriuretic factor (ANF). *Biochem. Biophys. Res. Commun.* 131: 1056–1062, 1985.
14. SCHWARTZ, D., D. M. GELLER, P. T. MANNING, N. R. SIEGEL, K. F. FOK, C. E. SMITH, AND

82   ATRIAL HORMONES AND OTHER NATRIURETIC FACTORS

P. NEEDLEMAN. Ser-Leu-Arg-Arg-atriopeptin III: the major circulating form of atrial peptide. *Science Wash. DC* 229: 397–400, 1985.

15. SEIDAH, N. G., C. LAZURE, M. CHRÉTIEN, G. THIBAULT, R. GARCIA, M. CANTIN, J. GENEST, R. F. NUTT, S. F. BRADY, T. A. LYLE, W. J. PALEVEDA, C. D. COLTON, T. M. CICCARONE, AND D. F. VEBER. Amino acid sequence of homologous rat atrial peptides: natriuretic activity of native and synthetic forms. *Proc. Natl. Acad. Sci. USA* 81: 2640–2644, 1984.

16. SEYMOUR, A. A., S. G. SMITH, E. K. MAZACK, AND E. H. BLAINE. A comparison of synthetic rat and human atrial natriuretic factor in conscious dogs. *Hypertension Dallas* 8: 211–216, 1986.

17. THIBAULT, G., R. GARCIA, M. CANTIN, J. GENEST, C. LAZURE, N. G. SEIDAH, AND M. CHRÉTIEN. Primary structure of a high Mr form of rat atrial natriuretic factor. *FEBS Lett.* 167: 352–356, 1984.

18. THIBAULT, G., R. GARCIA, F. CARRIER, N. G. SEIDAH, C. LAZURE, M. CHRÉTIEN, M. CANTIN, AND J. GENEST. Structure-activity relationships of atrial natriuretic factor (ANF). I. Natriuretic activity and relaxation of intestinal smooth muscle. *Biochem. Biophys. Res. Commun.* 125: 938–946, 1984.

19. THIBAULT, G., C. LAZURE, E. L. SCHIFFRIN, J. GUTKOWSKA, L. CHARTIER, R. GARCIA, N. G. SEIDAH, M. CHRÉTIEN, J. GENEST, AND M. CANTIN. Identification of a biologically active circulating form of rat atrial natriuretic factor. *Biochem. Biophys. Res. Commun.* 130: 981–986, 1985.

20. WAKITANI, K., M. G. CURRIE, D. M. GELLER, AND P. NEEDLEMAN. Vasodilator properties of a family of bioactive atrial peptides in isolated perfused rat kidneys. *J. Lab. Clin. Med.* 105: 349–352, 1985.

21. WAKITANI, K., T. OSHIMA, A. D. LOEWY, S. W. HOLMBERG, B. R. COLE, S. P. ADAMS, K. F. FOK, M. G. CURRIE, AND P. NEEDLEMAN. Comparative vascular pharmacology of the atriopeptins. *Circ. Res.* 56: 621–627, 1985.

22. WALDMAN, S. A., R. M. RAPOPORT, AND F. MURAD. Atrial natriuretic factor selectively activates particulate guanylate cyclase and elevates cyclic GMP in rat tissues. *J. Biol. Chem.* 259: 14332–14334, 1984.

8

Renal Actions of Atrial Natriuretic Peptides

BARBARA J. BALLERMANN, B. RENTZ DUNN,
RAMON E. MENDEZ, MARK L. ZEIDEL,
JULIAN L. SEIFTER, AND BARRY M. BRENNER

*Laboratory of Kidney and Electrolyte Physiology, Brigham and Women's Hospital
and Harvard Medical School, Boston, Massachusetts*

THE REPORT BY DE BOLD AND CO-WORKERS (11) of a dramatic increase in renal sodium and water excretion provoked by a natriuretic protein present in atrial extracts rapidly led to complete characterization of its peptide sequence (14) and gene structure (23). However, the mechanisms whereby atrial natriuretic peptides (ANP) augment renal sodium and water excretion are incompletely understood. The magnitude of the natriuresis that follows administration of ANP tends to suggest direct inhibition of renal sodium transport. Indeed, in early studies involving administration of atrial extracts in rats, Keeler and Azzarolo (19) reported increased sodium, potassium, phosphorus, magnesium, and calcium excretion and concluded that proximal tubule transport and possibly the transport functions of Henle's loop are inhibited by the atrial natriuretic factor. Also, Sonnenberg et al. (25) and Briggs and co-workers (6) suggested that the natriuretic action of atrial extracts is mediated, at least partly, by a direct effect of the atrial factor on distal sodium-transport functions. However, it is also evident from many studies that changes in renal hemodynamics play a significant role in the renal excretory response to ANP. In the isolated perfused kidney, ANP acted as a vasoconstrictor under baseline vasodilated conditions, whereas the peptide was clearly vasodilatory when infused in the presence of vasoconstrictors such as angiotensin II or norepinephrine (8). In whole-animal studies, transient ANP-induced increments in renal blood flow have been described by several investigators (15, 17, 20, 26, 27), and the glomerular filtration rate (GFR) has been observed to increase in many studies (4, 6, 7, 18, 20). Using the microsphere method, Borenstein et al. (5) observed a significant rise in inner cortical blood flow in response to atrial extract administration in the rat, while blood flow to the outer cortex decreased. Also, papillary plasma flow, determined by ^{125}I-labeled albumin

83

uptake, increased significantly within 5 min of atrial extract administration (5). Consequently it was suggested that alterations in medullary blood flow may have an important influence on the natriuretic response to ANP (5). Thus many studies have explored the renal actions of ANP. However, due to limitations in space, this chapter is concerned primarily with recent studies done in the authors' laboratories.

ROLE OF PERITUBULAR PHYSICAL FORCES

To address the role of hemodynamic factors in the renal response to ANP, the peptide was infused intravenously in rats, in the presence or absence of a suprarenal aortic clamp to reduce the renal perfusion pressure just enough to prevent an increase in GFR. The ANP augmented renal sodium excretion ~20-fold in rats with a normal renal perfusion pressure. In contrast, the response to ANP was almost completely abolished when renal perfusion pressure was reduced. These studies therefore suggest that enhanced renal sodium excretion in response to ANP cannot be accounted for solely by inhibition of renal tubule sodium transport. The dependence of the ANP-induced natriuretic response on adequate renal perfusion furthermore suggests that alterations in peritubular physical factors may be involved in eliciting the increase in renal sodium excretion. The alternative possibility, that the natriuresis results solely from the rise in GFR, although unlikely, is not ruled out. To delineate the potential role of changes in physical factors in the renal response to ANP, Mendez et al. (21) studied the influence of renal perfusion pressure and plasma oncotic pressure on ANP-induced renal sodium excretion. Infusion of ANP was associated with a fall in the mean arterial pressure from 111 ± 2 to 105 ± 2 mmHg (mean $\pm$ SE). When angiotensin II was administered in addition to ANP, mean arterial pressure rose to 121 ± 6 mmHg. Infusion of ANP alone increased the rate of renal sodium excretion to values 10-fold above base line; however, addition of angiotensin II during ANP infusion caused renal sodium excretion to increase even further, to 23-fold above base line. Angiotensin II and vehicle infusions raised renal sodium excretion only minimally. Alternatively, when rats were made hyperoncotic by exchange transfusion of 25% albumin for native plasma, the natriuretic response to ANP was nearly abolished. The magnitude of the increase in GFR was similar during infusion of ANP in isoncotic or hyperoncotic states and remained essentially unchanged during superimposition of angiotensin II compared with ANP infusion alone. Thus the increased natriuretic response to ANP with angiotensin II infusion and the marked decrease with hyperoncotic albumin could not be accounted for by changes in GFR (21). These data indicate that the elevation of peritubular capillary hydraulic pressure, by opposing reabsorption of tubule fluid, markedly augments the renal natriuretic response to ANP. Conversely, the presence of a high peritubular capillary oncotic pressure, which would tend to enhance reabsorption of tubule fluid, results in a pronounced blunting of renal sodium excretion in response to ANP. The data therefore support an important role for peritubular physical factors in the renal excretory response to ANP.

The renal hemodynamic effects of ANP were further delineated by micropuncture studies. At the glomerulus, ANP infusion produced a significant decrease in afferent and an increase in efferent arteriolar resistances, thus provoking a marked rise in glomerular capillary hydraulic pressure while the single-nephron plasma flow rate remained virtually constant (12). The net effect of these hemodynamic changes was a sharp increase in the single-nephron filtration fraction and an increase in the single-nephron GFR. The fall in afferent arteriolar resistance and the rise in glomerular capillary hydraulic pressure and efferent arteriolar resistance were found not to depend on the reduction in mean arterial pressure brought about by ANP infusion, thereby ruling out an indirect action of ANP on the glomerular microcirculation through alterations in systemic hemodynamics (12).

Assessment of Starling forces governing reabsorption of fluid from the proximal tubule showed that ANP infusion is associated with a rise in peritubular capillary oncotic pressure, as expected from the high filtration fraction, thereby tending to augment absolute proximal reabsorption. An increase in absolute proximal tubule fluid reabsorption (18) does not contradict findings of increased NaCl delivery out of the proximal tubule (6), as the filtered load of sodium increases markedly in response to ANP administration. Furthermore, fractional proximal reabsorption during ANP administration is reduced, indicating a degree of glomerulotubular imbalance (18). Although it has been suggested that ANP may affect transport mechanisms of the proximal tubule directly (16), in vitro perfusion of proximal tubule segments failed to show any direct effect of ANP on proximal tubule fluid reabsorption (3). Also, examination of microdissected nephron segments for specific ANP receptors showed that the proximal tubule is devoid of receptors for this hormone (9), making a direct action in this tubule segment doubtful.

Because ANP administration augments NaCl delivery to the last accessible portion of the superficial distal tubule by only ~2-fold (6), compared with the 10- to 50-fold increase in final urine sodium excretion usually observed (11), it is highly unlikely that alterations in glomerular hemodynamics and proximal reabsorption *alone* could account for the observed natriuresis. In addition, proximal events could not explain the ANP-induced rise in urinary sodium concentration to levels well above that of plasma, which Dunn et al. (13) observed. The marked increase in urinary sodium concentration in the presence of an increased urine flow rate suggests net addition of hypernatric interstitial fluid into the collecting duct lumen. Indeed, Sonnenberg et al. (25) previously provided evidence for an increase in absolute sodium delivery between outer medullary and papillary collecting ducts in response to atrial extract administration, suggesting addition of sodium to the luminal fluid of the papillary collecting duct. To assess possible alterations in papillary Starling forces in response to ANP, hydraulic pressures in the structures of the renal papilla were examined by Dunn and co-workers (13). Infusion of ANP resulted in raised hydraulic pressures within Henle's loop and in the inner medullary collecting duct but even more markedly in the descending and ascending vasa recta. Consequently the hydraulic pressure gradient between vasa recta and collecting duct increased with ANP infusion, an effect that would reduce vasa recta fluid uptake and thus fluid reabsorption from papillary collecting ducts.

PAPILLARY SODIUM CHLORIDE–TRANSPORT EFFECTS

The possibility of a direct action of ANP on the papillary collecting duct has also been explored. Studies by Zeidel and co-workers (29) showed that ANP significantly inhibits ouabain-sensitive oxygen consumption in a highly purified suspension of papillary collecting duct cells from the rabbit. This effect was not due to direct inhibition of Na^+-K^+-ATPase activity, as increasing sodium entry into cells by addition of the sodium ionophore amphotericin B augmented oxygen consumption equally in the presence or absence of ANP. It was therefore concluded that ANP inhibits sodium entry into papillary collecting duct cells, thereby indirectly reducing Na^+-K^+-ATPase activity. The inhibitory action of ANP on oxygen consumption was identical to the effect of amiloride, a known inhibitor of sodium entry in the collecting duct. The ANP had no effect on oxygen consumption in ascending limb or outer medullary collecting duct cells (29). Sodium-uptake studies with cultured monolayers of papillary collecting duct cells have since confirmed that ANP inhibits apical sodium entry in these cells (28). Finally, cGMP generation by papillary collecting duct cells is stimulated by ANP, and cGMP but not cAMP analogues mimic the effects of ANP on oxygen consumption in these cells (30). Thus it is logical to suggest that cGMP may be the second messenger that mediates the effect of ANP on sodium-transport–dependent oxygen consumption in papillary collecting duct cells.

SUMMARY OF MECHANISMS OF ANP ACTION IN THE KIDNEY

Taken together, the evidence argues for an interplay between renal hemodynamic and direct tubular actions of ANP. A proposed model of ANP action within the kidney is shown in Figure 1. At the glomerulus, afferent arteriolar dilatation in the presence of efferent arteriolar constriction brings about a rise in glomerular capillary hydraulic pressure (which leads to an increase in the filtration fraction) and a rise in GFR. The rise in filtration fraction contributes to an augmentation of absolute proximal fluid reabsorption, although not in proportion to the rise in GFR; accordingly, proximal fractional reabsorption decreases, leading to an increase of NaCl delivery out of the proximal tubule. Because ascending limb NaCl transport is not inhibited by ANP, enhanced NaCl delivery to this segment would tend to augment local transport and thereby addition of NaCl to the medullary interstitium. The high hydraulic pressures in the vasa recta would tend to diminish uptake of fluid from the medullary interstitium into the capillary lumen, thus leading to an accumulation of hypernatric papillary interstitial fluid. Although the rise

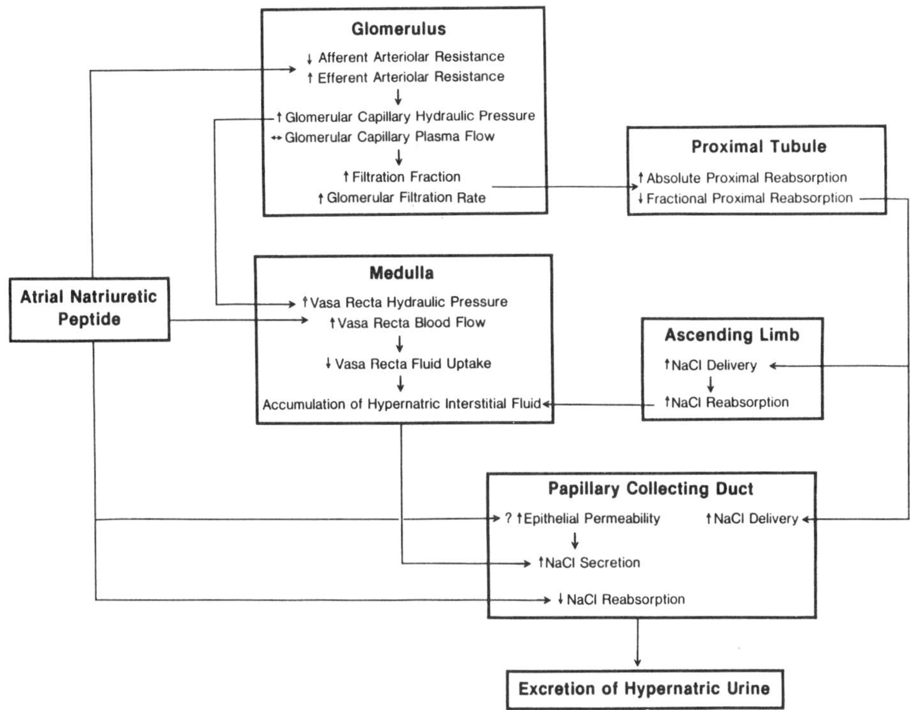

FIG. 1. Mechanisms whereby ANP leads to enhanced excretion of sodium-rich urine.

in vasa recta blood flow, which also accompanies ANP infusion (5), is thought to result in washout of the medullary osmotic gradient, Davis et al. (10) reported that the loss of medullary tonicity during ANP infusion was due primarily to a reduction in medullary urea content and not to a reduction in medullary NaCl concentration. The persistent concentration gradient for NaCl from medullary interstitium to collecting duct and the large hydraulic pressure gradient between vasa recta and papillary collecting duct would thus favor entry of NaCl and papillary interstitial fluid into the papillary collecting duct lumen. In addition, preliminary data by Rocha et al. (22) suggest that ANP enhances bath-to-lumen NaCl permeability in isolated rat papillary collecting ducts perfused in vitro, adding support to the possibility of enhanced NaCl uptake from medullary interstitium into papillary collecting ducts during ANP administration. In the presence of direct inhibition of NaCl reabsorption by ANP, excretion of hypernatric urine would thus be facilitated.

GLOMERULAR ANP RECEPTORS

In an effort to determine whether endogenous ANP plays a role in the day-to-day regulation of extracellular fluid volume (ECFV), studies were undertaken to evaluate potential target-tissue receptors for ANP in the kidney and to assess whether such receptors are regulated in response to changes in circulating concentrations of ANP. In isolated rat renal glomeruli, specific ANP receptors were demonstrated by radioligand binding techniques; ANP was found to markedly stimulate generation of cGMP, but not cAMP, in a concentration-dependent manner (2). Analogues of ANP that compete with high affinity for the glomerular receptor were also able to stimulate cGMP accumulation, whereas a physiologically inactive ANP analogue that does not bind to the receptor also did not stimulate the generation of cGMP. Thus the presence of specific, physiologically active ANP receptors in renal glomeruli was demonstrated. Cultured rat renal glomerular mesangial and epithelial cells were also studied to identify the glomerular cell type that expresses the ANP receptor. Cell surface receptors for ANP were found on glomerular mesangial cells but not on glomerular epithelial cells; cGMP generation was markedly enhanced by ANP only in the cells that contain receptors, namely the mesangial cells (2). As mesangial cells are thought to regulate blood flow within the glomerular microcirculation, these findings are consistent with a direct effect of ANP on glomerular hemodynamics. Whether ANP receptors are present on glomerular endothelial cells remains to be determined. To ascertain whether the glomerular ANP-receptor density is regulated by changes in circulating concentrations of ANP, plasma ANP levels and glomerular ANP-receptor density and affinity were determined in rats given furosemide (5 mg ip) and then fed a salt-deficient diet for 14 days. Rats were given either deionized water or isotonic saline solution to drink for the duration of the study (2). The glomerular ANP-receptor density was nearly fourfold higher in rats given no salt in their diet as compared with those given isotonic saline to drink. Although glomerular ANP-receptor density increased in salt-depleted rats, ANP-induced cGMP generation did not differ between glomeruli from rats given the low- versus the high-salt diet (Fig. 2), indicating that the glomerular ANP receptor may not be linked directly to guanylate cyclase. Plasma ANP concentrations were markedly higher in rats given saline to drink at 132 ± 63 compared with 23 ± 5 pM in rats given the salt-deficient diet alone. Thus the presence of specific, physiologically functional receptors in a renal target tissue for ANP and the reciprocal regulation of ANP-receptor density with changes in circulating ANP levels, brought about by alterations in dietary salt intake, suggest that endogenous ANP constitutes a hormonal system involved in ECFV regulation.

ANP SYSTEM DURING CHRONIC EXTRACELLULAR
FLUID VOLUME EXPANSION

Two chronic studies addressing the potential role of ANP in the regulation of sodium excretion have been performed. It is well known that the chronic administration of mineralocorticoid is associated with transient renal sodium retention followed by the return to neutral sodium balance, the so-called "escape" phenomenon. In rats given ~1 meq NaCl per day in their diet, sodium retention was observed during the first 24 h after injection of pharmacologic doses of deoxycorticosterone acetate (DOCA), followed, during the

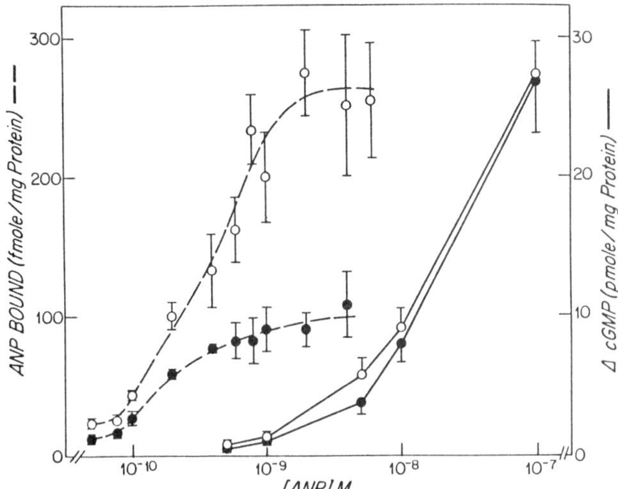

FIG. 2. Regulation of glomerular ANP-receptor density in salt-depleted (○) rats and rats fed a high-salt diet (●). At saturation, specific binding of ANP (– – – –) to glomeruli from salt-depleted rats was 4-fold higher than binding in glomeruli from high-salt rats, indicating a markedly lower ANP-receptor density in glomeruli from high-salt rats. ANP-induced cGMP generation (——) was unchanged despite the marked alteration in receptor density. Also, the concentrations of ANP required to stimulate cGMP generation in glomeruli are much higher than those associated with maximal binding to glomerular ANP receptors.

second 24-h period, by escape (1). Plasma ANP levels, determined by radioimmunoassay, rose nearly threefold at 12 and 24 h after DOCA administration and then returned to base line. Concomitant with the increase in plasma ANP levels, glomerular ANP-receptor density decreased, again suggesting regulation of receptor number by endogenous ANP. Furthermore, as plasma ANP concentrations rose, a marked increase in atrial preproANP mRNA content was observed, indicating a prompt rise in ANP gene transcription (1). These data indicate that DOCA administration in the rat is a powerful stimulus for ANP secretion. Whether ANP secretion was stimulated by DOCA directly, by DOCA-induced ECFV expansion, or by a combination of the two remains to be determined. Nevertheless, since ANP is a potent natriuretic agent, it is logical to propose that this hormone plays a role in initiating escape from the renal sodium-retaining effects of DOCA (1).

Smith et al. (24) recently explored the role of endogenous ANP in the adaptation to higher sodium excretion per nephron that regularly occurs in response to reduction in nephron number. Rats were subjected to five-sixths nephrectomy or sham operation and were placed on low-, normal-, or high-sodium intakes. Urinary sodium excretion rose with increasing dietary sodium intake in both groups, and sodium excretion per nephron was elevated in rats that were five-sixths nephrectomized as compared with control rats on the higher salt intakes. Plasma immunoreactive ANP did not change significantly with different sodium intake in sham-operated but rose progressively in five-sixths–nephrectomized rats with increasing sodium intake. Despite extensive nephron ablation, however, plasma ANP levels failed to rise in rats with reduced nephron number given a low-sodium diet, and in this group sodium excretion per nephron also failed to rise. These findings provide strong evidence that ANP plays an important role in promoting the adaptive increase in sodium excretion per nephron in chronic renal failure (24). Furthermore, restriction of dietary sodium in the setting of reduced GFR obviates the stimulation of ANP secretion as well as the adaptive increase in sodium excretion per nephron.

CONCLUSIONS

Within the kidney, ANP alters renal hemodynamics and thus peritubular physical forces governing fluid reabsorption, both at the level of the proximal tubule and in the renal papilla. In addition, ANP exerts a direct inhibitory effect on NaCl transport in the papillary collecting duct. It is proposed that the interplay between the actions of ANP on renal hemodynamics and papillary NaCl transport results in enhanced excretion of hypernatric urine. Specific ANP receptors are present in renal glomeruli and are localized, at least partly, on glomerular mesangial cells. Finally, the findings that the glomerular ANP-receptor density is regulated in response to alterations in circulating endogenous ANP, induced by changes in dietary salt intake; that ANP gene transcription and ANP secretion are augmented in response to mineralocorticoid-induced volume expansion; and that circulating ANP levels rise markedly in rats with reduced renal mass given a high-sodium intake, all indicate that ANP constitutes a hormonal system that responds to chronic changes in ECFV and probably participates in its regulation.

We thank Lynn Milburn for expert secretarial assistance.

This work was supported by grants from the National Institutes of Health (AM-35930) and Wyeth Laboratories.

REFERENCES

1. BALLERMANN, B. J., K. D. BLOCH, J. G. SEIDMAN, AND B. M. BRENNER. Atrial natriuretic peptide secretion, biosynthesis and glomerular receptor activity during mineralocorticoid escape. *J. Clin. Invest.* 78: 840–843, 1986.
2. BALLERMANN, B. J., R. L. HOOVER, M. J. KARNOVSKY, AND B. M. BRENNER. Physiologic regulation of atrial natriuretic peptide receptors in rat renal glomeruli. *J. Clin. Invest.* 76: 2049–2056, 1985.
3. BAUM, M., AND R. D. TOTO. Lack of a direct effect of atrial natriuretic factor in the rabbit proximal tubule. *Am. J. Physiol.* 250 (*Renal Fluid Electrolyte Physiol.* 19): F66–F69, 1986.
4. BEASLEY, D., AND R. L. MALVIN. Atrial extracts increase glomerular filtration rate in vivo. *Am. J. Physiol.* 248 (*Renal Fluid Electrolyte Physiol.* 17): F24–F30, 1985.
5. BORENSTEIN, H. B., W. A. CUPPLES, H. SONNENBERG, AND A. T. VERESS. The effect of a natriuretic atrial extract on renal haemodynamics and urinary excretion in anaesthetized rats. *J. Physiol. Lond.* 334: 133–140, 1983.
6. BRIGGS, J. P., B. STEIPE, G. SCHUBERT, AND J. SCHNERMANN. Micropuncture studies of the renal effects of atrial natriuretic substance. *Pfluegers Arch.* 395: 271–276, 1982.
7. BURNETT, J. C., JR., J. P. GRANGER, AND T. J. OPGENORTH. Effects of synthetic atrial

natriuretic factor on renal function and renin release. *Am. J. Physiol.* 247 (*Renal Fluid Electrolyte Physiol.* 16): F863–F866, 1984.

8. CAMARGO, M. J. F., H. D. KLEINERT, S. A. ATLAS, J. E. SEALEY, J. H. LARAGH, AND T. MAACK. Ca-dependent hemodynamic and natriuretic effects of atrial extract in isolated rat kidney. *Am. J. Physiol.* 246 (*Renal Fluid Electrolyte Physiol.* 15): F447–F456, 1984.

9. CANTIN, M., AND J. GENEST. The heart and the atrial natriuretic factor. *Endocr. Rev.* 6: 107–127, 1985.

10. DAVIS, C. L., J. SCHNERMANN, AND J. BRIGGS. Effect of atrial natriuretic factor on medullary solute gradients (abstr.). *Kidney Int.* 29: 414, 1986.

11. DE BOLD, A. J., H. B. BORENSTEIN, A. T. VERESS, AND H. SONNENBERG. A rapid and potent natriuretic response to intravenous injection of atrial myocardial extract in rats. *Life Sci.* 28: 89–94, 1981.

12. DUNN, B. R., I. ICHIKAWA, J. M. PFEFFER, J. L. TROY, AND B. M. BRENNER. Renal and systemic hemodynamic effects of synthetic atrial natriuretic peptide in the anesthetized rat. *Circ. Res.* 59: 237–246, 1986.

13. DUNN, B. R., J. L. TROY, I. ICHIKAWA, AND B. M. BRENNER. Effect of atrial natriuretic peptide (ANP) on hydraulic pressures in the rat renal papilla: implications for ANP-induced natriuresis. In: *Biologically Active Atrial Peptides. Proceedings of the First World Congress*, edited by B. M. Brenner and J. H. Laragh. New York: Raven, in press.

14. FLYNN, T. G., M. L. DE BOLD, AND A. J. DE BOLD. The amino acid sequence of an atrial peptide with potent diuretic and natriuretic properties. *Biochem. Biophys. Res. Commun.* 117: 859–865, 1983.

15. GARCIA, R., G. THIBAULT, J. GUTKOWSKA, M. CANTIN, AND J. GENEST. Changes of regional blood flow induced by atrial natriuretic factor (ANF) in conscious rats. *Life Sci.* 36: 1687–1692, 1985.

15. HAMMOND, T. G., A. N. K. YUSUFI, F. G. KNOX, AND T. P. DOUSA. Administration of atrial natriuretic factor inhibits sodium-coupled transport in proximal tubules. *J. Clin. Invest.* 75: 1983–1989, 1985.

17. HINTZE, T. H., M. G. CURRIE, AND P. NEEDLEMAN. Atriopeptins: renal-specific vasodilators in conscious dogs. *Am. J. Physiol.* 248 (*Heart Circ. Physiol.* 17): H587–H591, 1985.

18. HUANG, C. L., J. LEWICKI, L. K. JOHNSON, AND M. G. COGAN. Renal mechanism of action of rat atrial natriuretic factor. *J.Clin. Invest.* 75: 769–773, 1985.

19. KEELER, R., AND A. M. AZZAROLO. Effects of atrial natriuretic factor on renal handling of water and electrolytes in rats. *Can. J. Physiol. Pharmacol.* 61: 996–1002, 1983.

20. MAACK, T., D. N. MARION, M. J. CAMARGO, H. D. KLEINERT, J. H. LARAGH, E. D. VAUGHAN, JR., AND S. A. ATLAS. Effect of auriculin (atrial natriuretic factor) on blood pressure, renal function, and the renin-aldosterone system in dogs. *Am. J. Med.* 77: 1069–1075, 1984.

21. MENDEZ, R. E., B. R. DUNN, J. L. TROY, AND B. M. BRENNER. Modulation of the natriuretic response to atrial natriuretic peptide by alterations in peritubular starting forces. *Circ. Res.* In press.

22. ROCHA, A. S., L. H. KUDO, AND T. MAACK. Acao do fator atrial Na absorcao de NaCl e H20 do ducto coletor papilar (abstr.). In: *Proc. Congr. Latino Americano Nefrologia, 6th, Rio de Janeiro, Brazil, October, 1985*, p. 76.

23. SEIDMAN, S. E., K. D. BLOCH, K. A. KLEIN, J. A. SMITH, AND J. G. SEIDMAN. Nucleotide sequences of the human and mouse atrial natriuretic factor genes. *Science Wash. DC* 226: 1206–1209, 1984.

24. SMITH, S., S. ANDERSON, B. J. BALLERMANN, AND B. M. BRENNER. Role of atrial natriuretic peptide in the adaptation of sodium excretion with reduced renal mass. *J. Clin. Invest.* 77: 1395–1398, 1986.

25. SONNENBERG, H., W. A. CUPPLES, A. J. DE BOLD, AND A. T. VERESS. Intrarenal localization of the natriuretic effect of cardiac atrial extract. *Can. J. Physiol. Pharmacol.* 60: 1149–1152, 1982.

26. WAKITANI, K., B. R. COLE, D. M. GELLER, M. G. CURRIE, S. P. ADAMS, K. F. FOK, AND P. NEEDLEMAN. Atriopeptins: correlation between renal vasodilation and natriuresis. *Am. J. Physiol.* 249 (*Renal Fluid Electrolyte Physiol.* 18): F49–F53, 1985.

27. WAKITANI, K., T. OSHIMA, A. D. LOEWY, S. W. HOLMBERG, B. R. COLE, S. P. ADAMS, K. F. FOK, M. G. CURRIE, AND P. NEEDLEMAN. Comparative vascular pharmacology of the atriopeptins. *Circ. Res.* 56: 621–627, 1985.

28. ZEIDEL, M. L., J. L. SEIFTER, B. M. BRENNER, AND S. SARIBAN-SOHRABY. Atrial natriuretic peptide and amiloride inhibit apical Na$^+$ flux in cultured rabbit inner medullary collecting

duct cells. In: *Biologically Active Atrial Peptides. Proceedings of the First World Congress*, edited by B. M. Brenner and J. H. Laragh. New York: Raven, in press.
29. ZEIDEL, M. L., J. L. SEIFTER, S. LEAR, B. M. BRENNER, AND P. SILVA. Atrial peptides inhibit oxygen consumption in kidney medullary collecting duct cells. *Am. J. Physiol.* 251 (*Renal Fluid Electrolyte Physiol.* 20): F379–F383, 1986.
30. ZEIDEL, M. L., P. SILVA, B. M. BRENNER, AND J. L. SEIFTER. Role of cGMP in atrial natriuretic peptide (ANP) inhibition of Na$^+$ transport by rabbit inner medullary collecting duct cells. In: *Biologically Active Atrial Peptides. Proceedings of the First World Congress*, edited by B. M. Brenner and J. H. Laragh. New York: Raven, in press.

9

Effect of Atrial Peptides on the Adrenal Cortex

PATRICK J. MULROW, ROBERTO FRANCO-SAENZ,
K. ATARASHI, MASAO TAKAGI, AND MARI TAKAGI

Department of Medicine, Medical College of Ohio, Toledo, Ohio

EARLIER STUDIES ON THE CONTROL of aldosterone secretion suggested that an inhibitory system also regulates secretion. In 1958 Mills et al. (22) reported increased aldosterone secretion in dogs during constriction of the inferior vena cava; when the constriction was released, the aldosterone secretion rate fell below the basal level. Resection of the cervical vagi did not affect the increase in secretion but prevented the decrease. In 1959 Anderson et al. (2) reported that stretching of the right atria inhibited aldosterone secretion in the dog. Other studies (11, 16) also supported an inhibitory system of aldosterone production. Through the years this inhibition was thought to be due to an unknown central reflex mechanism.

INHIBITION OF ANGIOTENSIN II, POTASSIUM, AND ACTH STIMULATION OF ALDOSTERONE PRODUCTION BY ATRIAL NATRIURETIC FACTOR (ANF)

In Vitro Inhibition

In view of the data supporting regulation of aldosterone secretion by an inhibitory system and the demonstration of biological activity in atrial extracts, we investigated the effect of crude atrial extracts on aldosterone production by the rat adrenal gland. We used dispersed glomerulosa and fasciculata cells in vitro (5). Briefly, the rat adrenal glands are removed, defatted, and the capsular cells separated by standard techniques. These cells contain primarily glomerulosa cells and are ~95% pure; the inner zone contains fascicular-medullary cells. Incubation is carried out in medium 199 with or

93

without addition of various stimulators. Aldosterone is measured in the media as an index of steroid production by the glomerulosa cells, and corticosterone is measured as an index of production by the fasciculata cells. Initially we used crude rat atrial extracts. This was before synthetic peptides were available.

The effect of a crude atrial extract on the basal production of aldosterone by capsular cells of the zona glomerulosa is shown in Figure 1. The dilution of the extract and amount of protein in each dilution is shown on the abscissa. The atrial extract inhibits aldosterone production in a dose-dependent fashion, whereas extracts of ventricular muscle have no effect. The crude atrial extract also has diuretic and natriuretic activity when injected into rats. The activity of these extracts is destroyed by incubation with trypsin, and furthermore there is no evidence the extracts damage the adrenal cells, since the cells are able to exclude trypan blue dye.

The atrial extract inhibits the stimulation of aldosterone by ACTH (Fig. 2). The ACTH stimulates aldosterone production in a dose-dependent manner. The addition of the atrial extract to the ACTH incubation markedly lowers the basal aldosterone production and shifts the ACTH dose-response curve to the right. However, higher doses of ACTH overcome the inhibition, and the maximal stimulation by ACTH (with or without the addition of the atrial extract) is approximately the same. Also shown in Figure 2 is the dose-response

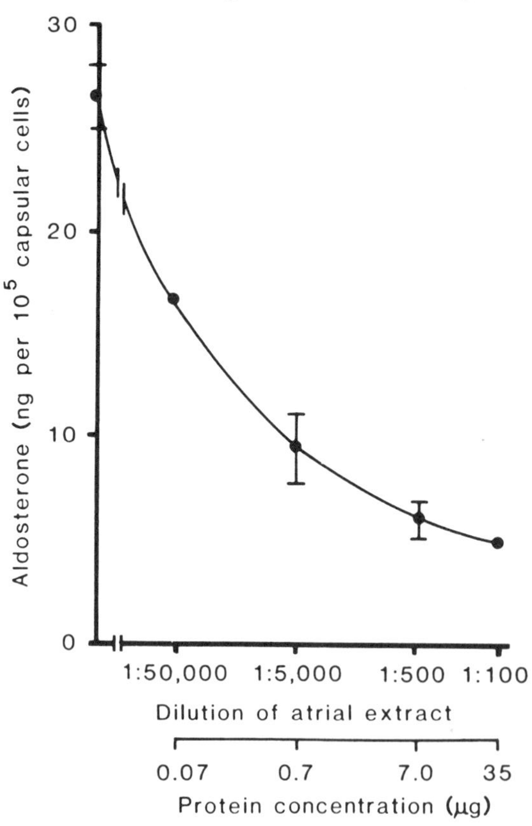

FIG. 1. Inhibition of secretion of aldosterone from unstimulated capsular cells by an atrial extract. Point without atrial extract and points of 1:5,000 and 1:500 dilution of extract each represent mean ± SE of 5 experiments. Other 2 points show mean of duplicate incubations in 1 experiment. One milliliter of incubation medium 199 contained a final dilution of atrial extract as indicated by the abscissa. Immediately beneath the dilution is amount of atrial extract protein that was added to 1 ml of incubation medium for a given dilution. [From Atarashi et al. (5).]

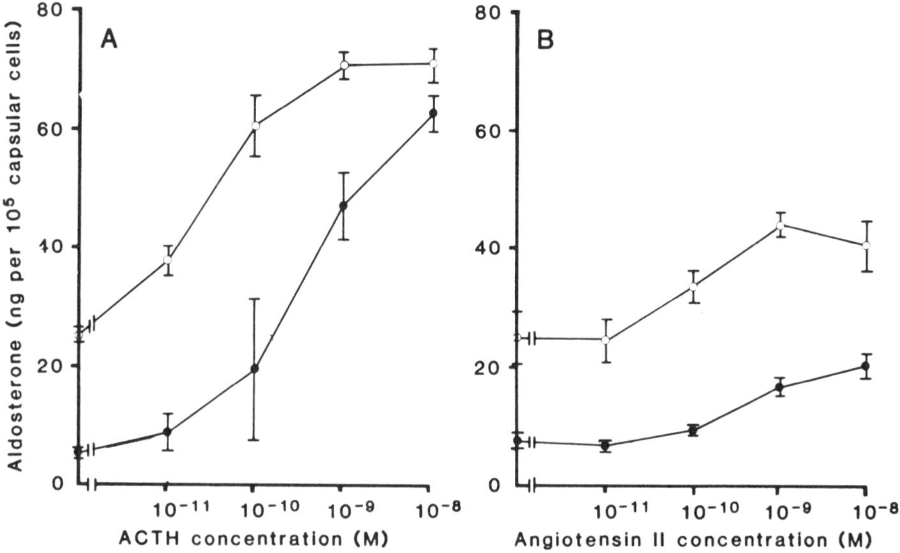

FIG. 2. *A*: aldosterone production by ACTH with atrial extract (●; 1:500 dilution) and without atrial extract (○). Each point represents mean ± SE of 5 separate experiments. ACTH concentrations are expressed as moles per liter of incubation medium. *B*: aldosterone production by angiotensin II with atrial extract (●; 1:500 dilution) and without atrial extract (○). Each point represents mean ± SE of 3 experiments. Angiotensin II concentrations are expressed as moles per liter of incubation medium. [From Atarashi et al. (5).]

curve of aldosterone production to angiotensin II. As the dose of angiotensin II increases, aldosterone production increases, reaching a maximum at 10^{-9} M. When atrial extract is added to the angiotensin incubation, there is a decrease in the basal production of aldosterone and an inhibition of the response to angiotensin II. In contrast to ACTH, higher doses of angiotensin II cannot overcome the inhibition by the extract. The atrial extract has no effect on corticosterone production by fasciculata cells, either in the basal state or in response to ACTH stimulation.

With the availability of synthetic peptides, we studied the effect of atriopeptin I (the 21–amino acid peptide), atriopeptin II (the 23–amino acid peptide), and atriopeptin III (the 24–amino acid peptide) (3, 4). All three atriopeptins significantly inhibit aldosterone production (Fig. 3). Atriopeptin II and III are more potent than atriopeptin I. This latter finding is similar to the report of Campbell et al. (7), who showed that atriopeptin III was more potent than atriopeptin I in inhibiting aldosterone production. The effect of atriopeptin II on aldosterone production stimulated by ACTH is depicted in Figure 4. The addition of 10 nmol atriopeptin II inhibits the basal level of aldosterone and shifts the dose-response curve to the right. With the higher doses of ACTH, the inhibition is overcome. This dose-response curve is similar to that observed with the crude atrial extract. The effect of atriopeptin II on aldosterone production stimulated by angiotensin II is shown in Figure 5. There is a significant increase in aldosterone production in response to

FIG. 3. Inhibition of aldosterone secretion in unstimulated capsular cells by atriopeptin I, II, and III. Each point represents mean ± SE of 4–6 experiments done in duplicate. Ap I, $n = 4$; Ap II, $n = 6$; Ap III, $n = 4$ (n, number of experiments). Atriopeptin concentrations are expressed as moles per liter of incubation medium. Asterisks, values significantly different from control value: $*P < 0.005$; $**P < 0.01$; $***P < 0.001$. Significance calculated by one-way analysis of variance and Scheffe's multiple-range analysis. [From Atarashi et al. (4).]

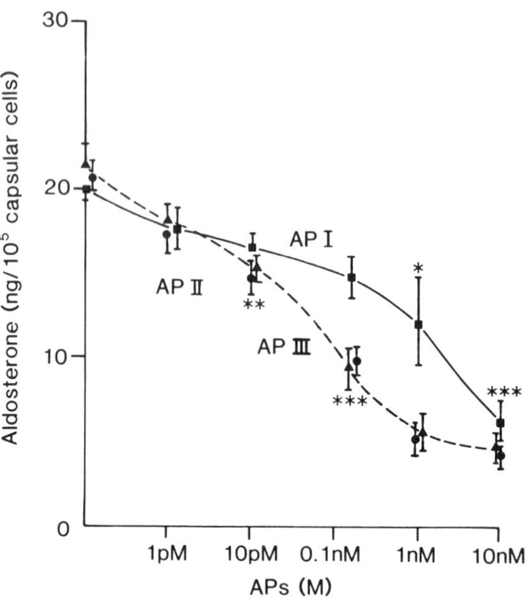

FIG. 4. Effect of atriopeptin II (Ap II) on aldosterone production elicited by ACTH. Each point represents mean ± SE of 6 experiments done in duplicate, except where indicated by †, where number of experiments is 3. In each experiment, ACTH concentrations are expressed as moles per liter of incubation medium. [From Atarashi et al. (4).]

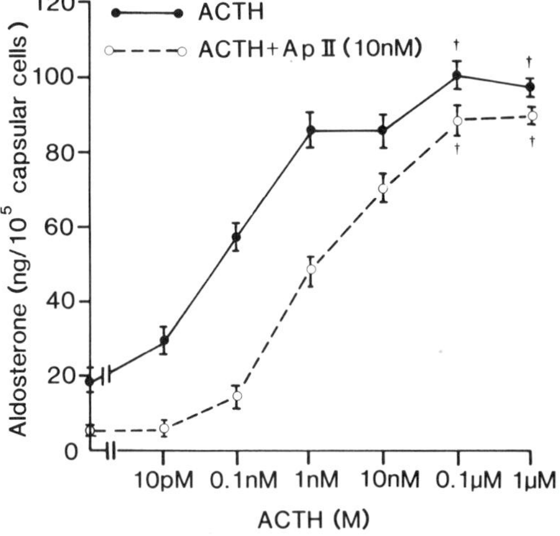

angiotensin II. However, when atriopeptin II is added at 10 nmol, basal production is diminished and the response to angiotensin II is markedly diminished. Even high doses of angiotensin II cannot overcome the inhibition by atriopeptin. These results are similar to those seen with the crude atrial extract.

The inhibition of steroidogenesis by atriopeptin is specific for the zona glomerulosa in the rat. Corticosterone production is increased in a dose-dependent fashion by ACTH stimulation of fasciculata cells. Atriopeptin II does not inhibit the basal production of corticosterone nor the stimulation by ACTH (Fig. 6). In cultured bovine adrenal cells, there is some evidence that atriopeptins can inhibit production of cortisol by fasciculata cells (10). How-

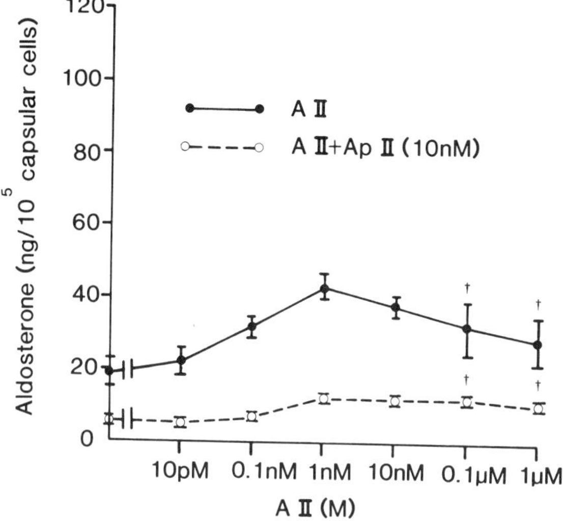

FIG. 5. Effect of atriopeptin II (Ap II) on aldosterone production elicited by angiotensin II (A II). Each point represents mean ± SE of 5 experiments done in duplicate, except where indicated by †, where number of experiments is 2. Angiotensin II concentrations are expressed as moles per liter of incubation medium. [From Atarashi et al. (4).]

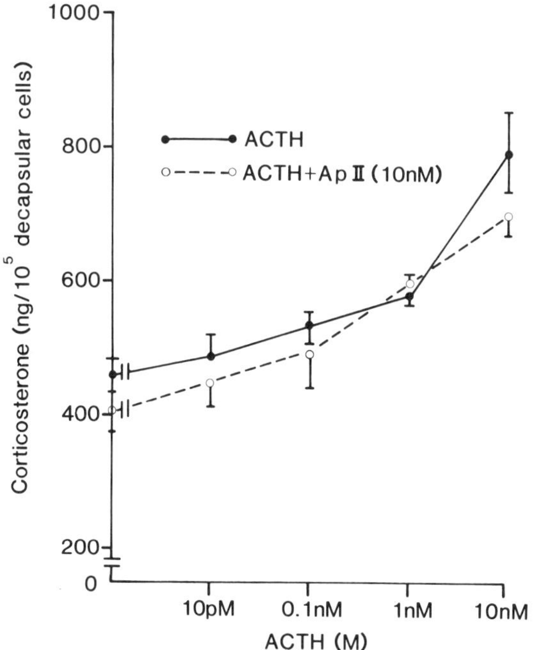

FIG. 6. Effect of atriopeptin II (Ap II) on basal and ACTH-stimulated corticosterone production by fasciculata cells. Each point represents mean ± SE of 5–6 experiments done in duplicate. [From Atarashi et al. (4).]

ever, the bovine cell is different from the human and the rat cell in that bovine fasciculata cells also respond to angiotensin stimulation with an increase in cortisol.

In Vivo Inhibition

The next series of experiments was designed to determine if atriopeptins could inhibit aldosterone response in vivo. We studied the effect of infusion of atriopeptins in conscious female Sprague-Dawley rats weighing ~200 g and eating a normal-sodium diet. The methodology has been described previously (3); briefly, polyethylene catheters are implanted into the right common carotid and internal jugular vein, ~48 h before the experiment. The catheters are led subcutaneously to the back of the neck, exteriorized, and filled with heparinized saline to keep patent. Two hours before the experiment the rats are given dexamethasone phosphate, 1 mg/kg intraperitoneally, to inhibit release of ACTH during the experiment. At zero time a small amount of blood is taken from the carotid catheter and the blood loss is replaced with the same volume of isotonic saline. Subsequently, angiotensin 0.2 $nmol \cdot kg^{-1} \cdot min^{-1}$, is infused continuously through the jugular catheter with or without an infusion of atriopeptin II at the rate of either 1 $nmol \cdot kg^{-1} \cdot min^{-1}$ or 2 $nmol \cdot kg^{-1} \cdot min^{-1}$ for 30 min. Plasma aldosterone is measured before and after the infusion. Plasma renin activity (PRA), corticosterone, potassium, and hematocrit are determined at the end of the infusion.

The effect of simultaneous infusion of atriopeptin II and angiotensin on plasma aldosterone is graphed in Figure 7. Angiotensin markedly increases plasma aldosterone levels. When atriopeptin II is infused simultaneously with angiotensin, there is a marked suppression of the response to angiotensin II. The multiple variables that were measured at the end of the infusion are shown in Table 1. Although atriopeptin II markedly inhibits the aldosterone response to angiotensin, there is no effect on serum corticosterone, potassium, or PRA levels. The hematocrit is increased by the infusion of atriopeptin. This

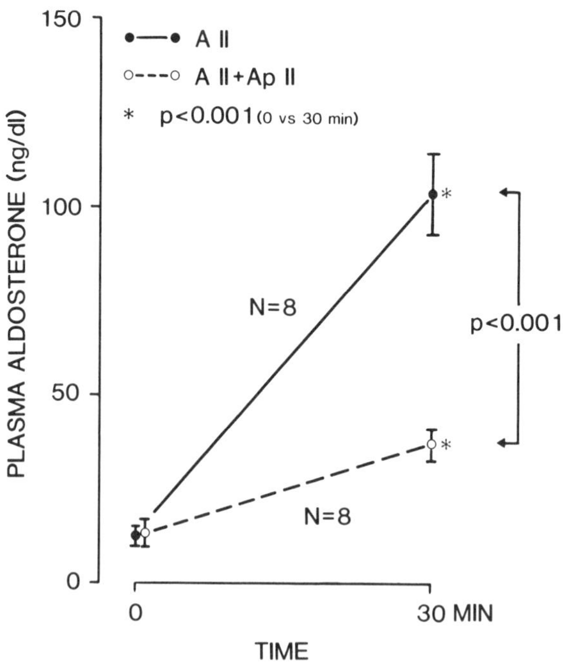

FIG. 7. In vivo inhibition by atriopeptin II (Ap II) of plasma aldosterone stimulated by angiotensin II (A II). Angiotensin II was infused either alone or with atriopeptin II. Ordinate, plasma aldosterone; abscissa, time of infusion. *n*, Number of rats studied in each group. [From Atarashi et al. (4).]

TABLE 1. *Effect of infusions of angiotension II or angiotensin II plus atriopeptin II on plasma levels of aldosterone, corticosterone, potassium, PRA, and hematocrit*

	Angiotensin II	Angiotensin II plus Atriopeptin II	P
Aldosterone, ng/dl	98.50 ± 19.40	33.80 ± 5.10	<0.02
Corticosterone, μg/dl	3.98 ± 1.99	5.67 ± 1.31	
Potassium, meq/liter	3.75 ± 0.14	3.83 ± 0.05	
PRA, ng AI·ml^{-1}·h^{-1}	9.5 ± 4.85	12.9 ± 3.64	
Hematocrit, %	46.60 ± 0.89	50.90 ± 0.48	<0.01

Results were obtained at end of 30-min infusions (mean ± SE) in 4 rats in each group. PRA, plasma renin activity.

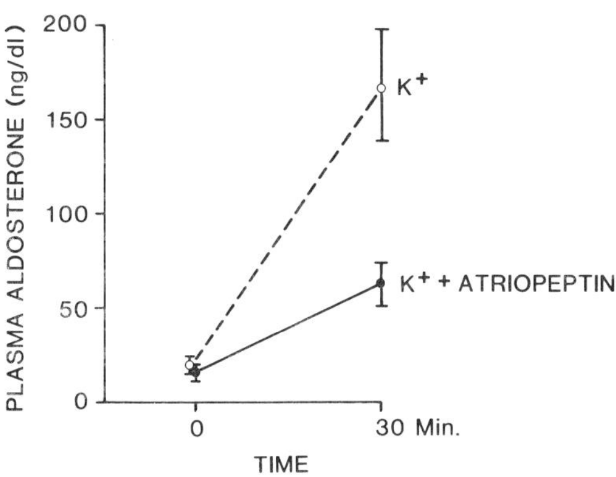

FIG. 8. Plasma aldosterone levels before and after infusion of 0.08 meq· kg^{-1}·min^{-1} potassium (o– – –o) or 0.08 meq·kg^{-1}·min^{-1} potassium with atriopeptin II (●——●). Each point represents mean ± SE. [From Takagi et al. (26).]

increase is due in part to the diuresis and in part to the now-recognized increase in capillary permeability that occurs with atriopeptide infusions.

We then studied the effect of atriopeptin on the stimulation of aldosterone production by infusions of potassium. A potassium chloride solution was infused at the rate of 0.08 meq·kg^{-1} body wt·min^{-1} through the jugular vein to one group of six rats for 30 min.

The second group received an infusion of atriopeptin II at the concentration of 0.2 nmol·kg^{-1}·min^{-1} for 30 min along with the infusion of potassium chloride. The potassium chloride infusion alone causes a marked stimulation of plasma aldosterone within 30 min. In contrast, the atriopeptin II infused simultaneously with potassium markedly blunts this response to potassium (Fig. 8). The plasma potassium levels are not significantly different between the two groups. In the group that received only potassium, the serum potassium at the end of the infusion reaches a level of 6.52 ± 0.30 meq/liter (mean ± SE), whereas the level when both atriopeptin II and potassium were infused was 6.0 ± 0.16 meq/liter. The PRA and corticosterone levels are also similar between the two groups. It appears that atriopeptin II blocked the stimulation of aldosterone by potassium at the adrenal level (26).

It is clear, therefore, that atriopeptin II can inhibit the effect of exogenous stimuli on aldosterone production. We next studied the effect of infusions of atriopeptin III on basal aldosterone production in vivo in rats maintained on a normal-sodium diet. These rats were conscious, unrestrained, and infused with either isotonic saline or atriopeptin III, as in the previous experiments.

EFFECT OF ANF ON RENIN RELEASE IN VIVO AND IN VITRO

The results of low and high doses of ANF on the levels of PRA and plasma aldosterone are shown in Table 2. Two different doses of atriopeptin III were infused. Plasma aldosterone was measured before the infusion and also at the end of the infusion. The PRA was measured at the end of the infusion. In the saline control the plasma aldosterone is 17 ng/dl, which is the usual finding in unrestrained rats on a normal-sodium diet. At the end of the saline infusion, it is slightly decreased at 11.7 ng/dl. When the dose of atriopeptide is infused at 5×10^{-11} mol·kg^{-1}·min^{-1}, the aldosterone levels and PRA values are unchanged from the control. In contrast, when a higher dose of ANF is used (0.2 nmol·kg^{-1}·min^{-1}), there is a significant increase in PRA at the end of the infusion, and aldosterone is increased from the preinfusion level of 17 to 22 ng/dl after the infusion. This is significantly different from the saline control rats, which showed a value of 11.7 ng/dl at the end of the infusion (27).

In separate experiments the high dose of ANF was shown to cause hypotension in the rat, reducing the blood pressure by ~10–20 mmHg. Presumably this high dose, by indirectly causing hypotension, increased renin secretion. Also, there is an increase in corticosterone level, presumably due to a release of ACTH as a result of the hypotension. These two effects, high renin and high ACTH, may offset any inhibition of atriopeptide on aldosterone production. The results in the literature on the effect of atriopeptin infusions in vivo on renin production in either rat, dog, or human are conflicting.

A summary of the results of infusion of ANF on renin and aldosterone production in vivo in rats is shown in Table 3. In addition to the results previously shown in Table 2, Takagi et al. (27) and Chartier et al. (9) reported that in the basal condition there was no effect on PRA or on plasma aldosterone

TABLE 2. *Effect of low- and high-dose ANF on levels of PRA and plasma aldosterone*

	Saline Alone	Low-Dose ANF	High-Dose ANF
Plasma aldosterone			
Before infusion, ng/dl	17.3 ± 1.8	20.5 ± 3.4	17.0 ± 2.6
After infusion, ng/dl	11.7 ± 0.5	12.4 ± 1.0	22.3 ± 1.4*
PRA after infusion, ng AI·ml^{-1}·h^{-1}	2.51 ± 0.37	3.43 ± 0.61	8.20 ± 1.48*
Plasma corticosterone, μg/dl	0.58 ± 0.07	1.56 ± 0.81	5.04 ± 1.22*
Plasma potassium, meq/liter	3.83 ± 0.08	3.86 ± 0.08	3.80 ± 0.10

Low-dose atrial natriuretic factor (ANF) did not affect plasma renin activity (PRA) or plasma aldosterone. High-dose ANF significantly increased PRA, plasma aldosterone, and corticosterone. Low-dose ANF, bolus 5×10^{-10} mol/kg + 5×10^{-11} mol·kg^{-1}·min^{-1} for 30 min. High-dose ANF, bolus 5×10^{-9} mol/kg + 5×10^{-10} mol·kg^{-1}·min^{-1} for 30 min. Values are means ± SE.   *$P < 0.01$ compared with saline alone. No significant difference in any of the parameters when saline alone was compared with low-dose ANF.

TABLE 3. *Effect of ANF on PRA and aldosterone production in vivo in rat*

Condition	PRA	Aldosterone	Ref.
Basal	0	0	27
	0	0	9
2K-1C	↓		16
	↑	↓	29
1K-1C	0		15
	0	0	29
1K-1C-LS	↓	↓	29

Basal, conscious unrestrained rats with chronic catheters. PRA, plasma renin activity. 0, no change. 2K-1C, rats with hypertension due to clip on renal artery of one kidney. 1K-1C, rats with hypertension due to clip on renal artery of remaining kidney. 1K-1C-LS, same as 1K-1C, except rats were on a low-sodium diet.

TABLE 4. *Effect of ANF on PRA and aldosterone in vivo*

Condition	PRA	Aldosterone	Ref.
Dog			
Anesthetized	↓	↓	20
	↓		6
	0		25
Conscious	0	0	13
Caval constricted*	↓	↓	13
Human			
Essential hypertension	0	↓	24
Basal†	0	0	28
	0	0	31
	0	↓	30
High-, normal-, low-sodium diet‡	↑	↓	32

* Thoracic inferior vena cava was constricted. † Resting, conscious, normal subjects on a normal-sodium diet. ‡ Normal subjects on a high-, normal-, or low-sodium diet; 3 groups responded in same direction.

levels. In the two-kidney, one clip rat with hypertension, Garcia et al. (16) gave ANF by chronic minipump infusion and measured a fall in the elevated PRA. However, in the one-kidney, one clip hypertensive rat, these same authors showed no effect on PRA (15). Aldosterone was not measured in these experiments. Volpe et al. (29) infused ANF into the two-kidney, one clip hypertensive rat, which resulted in an increase in PRA and a decrease in aldosterone. In the one-kidney, one clip hypertensive rat, the ANF infusion had no effect on renin or aldosterone. However, when the one-kidney, one clip rat was placed on a low-sodium diet, the rats developed an angiotensin-dependent type of hypertension and infusion of ANF decreased both PRA and aldosterone.

The effect of ANF administration in both dog and human is shown in Table 4. The experiment by Maack et al. (20) shows that in the anesthetized dog there is a decrease in PRA and a decrease in plasma aldosterone. Burnett et al. (6) infused a large dose of ANF into the renal artery of anesthetized dogs and showed a significant decrease in renin secretion. Seymour et al. (25) also infused ANF into the renal artery of anesthetized dogs at a somewhat lower dose than did Burnett et al. and showed no effect on renin secretion. Freeman et al. (13) infused ANF into the conscious dog under basal conditions and reported no effect on the PRA or plasma aldosterone. In contrast, when they infused the same dose into dogs with caval constriction and very high levels of circulating renin and aldosterone, there was a decrease in both PRA and aldosterone. The results in humans are somewhat conflicting. Richards et al. (24) gave a bolus injection of synthetic ANF; this had no effect on PRA but caused a decrease in aldosterone. Tikkanen et al. (28) infused ANF into normal humans under basal conditions and found no effect on PRA or aldosterone, although there was a trend toward lower PRA values during the infusion. Weidmann et al. (31) infused ANF into normal humans under basal conditions while they were on a normal-sodium diet; despite a hypotensive effect of the peptide, there was no change in PRA or plasma aldosterone. In a more extensive study, Weidmann et al. (32) reported an increase in PRA during infusion in normal humans on either a high-, normal-, or low-sodium diet. Plasma aldosterone levels were diminished. Despite 6 h of infusion of α-human atrial natriuretic peptide (α-hANP) into 6 normal humans on a high-sodium intake, Waldhausel et al. (30) reported no change in PRA but a lowering of plasma aldosterone. It appears, therefore, that the effect of infusion of ANF on PRA changes with the experimental condition. When PRA and aldosterone are simultaneously suppressed, it is difficult to interpret whether the effect of the ANF is directly on the adrenal to inhibit aldosterone or is inhibiting aldosterone by lowering renin secretion. However, plasma aldosterone is more consistently reduced than PRA; the evidence favors a direct inhibition by ANF on the adrenal gland in vivo. The effect on renin production is less consistent, with values going either up or down. The reports of a direct effect in vitro on kidney slices are also conflicting. Experiments by Obana et al. (23) suggest a direct inhibition of ANF on renin release in vitro. In contrast, our group has been unable to demonstrate an inhibition of ANF on renin release by superfused rat kidney slices in vitro, either in the basal state or after stimulation by isoproterenol (Figs. 9 and 10; 27).

MECHANISM OF INHIBITION OF ALDOSTERONE PRODUCTION BY ANF

The mechanism by which ANF inhibits aldosterone production at the adrenal level is not clear. Several of the biosynthetic steps by which steroidogenesis is stimulated by a variety of stimuli are understood. The ACTH binds to a plasma membrane receptor and activates adenylate cyclase, generating cAMP, which in turn leads to a series of steps that results in the production of a labile protein that enhances the conversion of cholesterol to pregnenolone. Angiotensin II has its own specific membrane receptor, while the initial event in potassium stimulation is depolarization of the cell membrane. All three stimuli enhance production of this labile protein, which enhances the entrance of cholesterol to the inner mitochondrial membrane where it is converted to

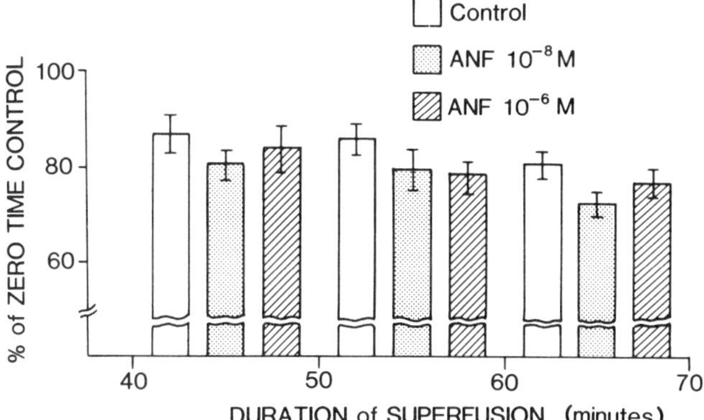

FIG. 9. Rat kidney slices were superfused with Krebs-Ringer-bicarbonate buffer. Zero time control, i.e., the 0- to 10-min renin release for each slice, after the washout period, is represented as 100% on ordinate. Duration of superfusion, time of superfusion of each slice from zero time. Height of bar in each time period, renin release as percent of zero time control. Each kidney slice served as its own control. Release of renin from control slice decreased slightly with time. ANF did not inhibit basal renin release. □, Buffer superfusing kidney slice had a concentration of atriopeptin III of 10^{-8} M; ▨, concentration of atriopeptin III of 10^{-6} M.

pregnenolone. Inhibitors of protein synthesis will inhibit the action of ACTH, angiotensin II, or potassium on aldosterone production.

Biosynthetic Pathway

Figure 11 is a diagram of the biosynthetic pathway of aldosterone in the zona glomerulosa. The early step is the conversion of cholesterol to pregnenolone. This is the rate-limiting step controlled by the labile protein. Goodfriend et al. (17) and later Campbell et al. (7) reported that the cholesterol-to-pregnenolone step is inhibited by ANF.

Goodfriend et al. (17) used bovine adrenal cells and synthetic 24–amino acid ANF (which they called auriculin) to inhibit pregnenolone production and thus block the early pathway. These authors also used a more-polar cholesterol derivative, 25-hydroxycholesterol, which enters the mitochondria more easily than cholesterol. Passage through the inner mitochondrial membrane is thought to be the rate-limiting step. The increment in aldosterone production induced by the addition of 25-hydroxycholesterol acetate was unaffected by ANF. Campbell et al. (7) showed that in addition to the block in the early pathway, there is inhibition of the late pathway, conversion of corticosterone to aldosterone.

Plasma Membrane Binding, cAMP, cGMP

Other steps involved in the action of ANF have been worked out. De Léan et al. (10) have demonstrated specific binding sites for ANF on adrenal

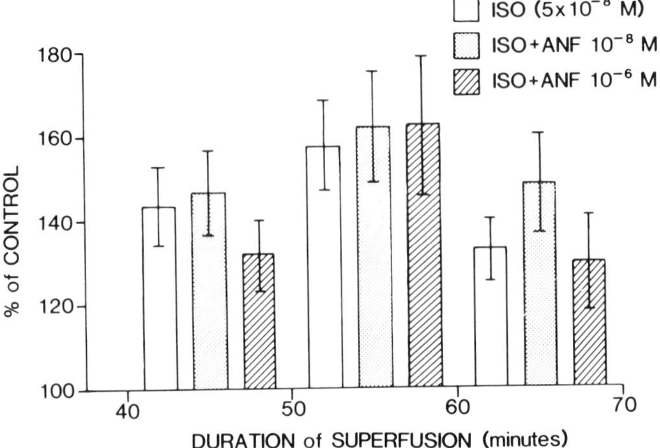

FIG. 10. Rat kidney slices were perfused with Krebs-Ringer-bicarbonate buffer. Zero time control, i.e., the 0- to 10-min renin release for each slice, after the washout period, is represented as 100% on ordinate. Duration of superfusion, time of superfusion of each slice from zero time. Height of bar in each time period, renin release as percent of zero time control. Each kidney slice served as its own control. ANF did not inhibit isoproterenol-induced renin release. □, Isoproterenol alone (which stimulated renin release over control levels ~200%). ▨ and ▧, Simultaneous superfusion of isoproterenol and ANF.

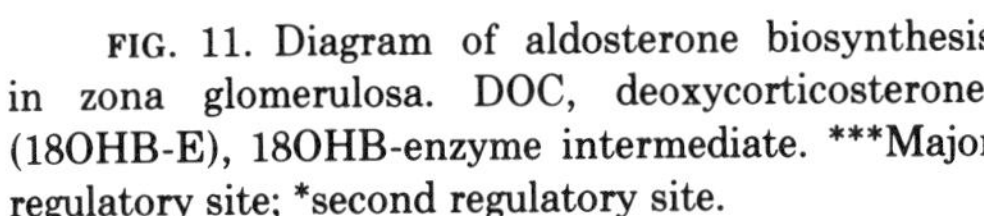

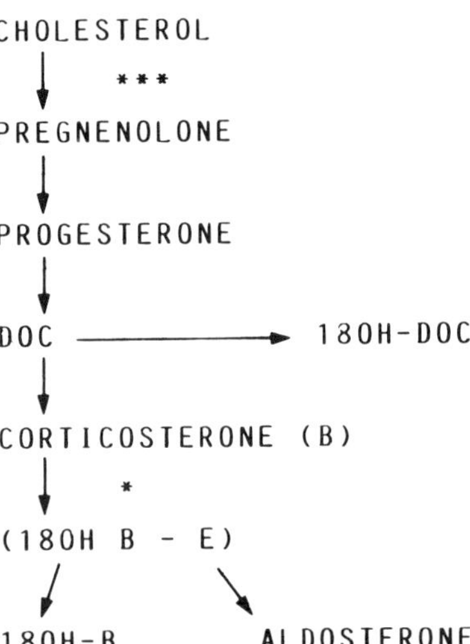

FIG. 11. Diagram of aldosterone biosynthesis in zona glomerulosa. DOC, deoxycorticosterone. (18OHB-E), 18OHB-enzyme intermediate. ***Major regulatory site; *second regulatory site.

membranes. The ANF has a high-affinity site on the adrenal membrane and is readily displaced by ANF but not by angiotensin II or ACTH. Furthermore, ANF does not displace angiotensin II from its binding sites. Thus ANF has a specific binding site on the plasma membrane of the zona glomerulosa cell that is separate from the receptors for ACTH and angiotensin II.

Anand-Srivastava et al. (1) have shown that ANF inhibits adenylate

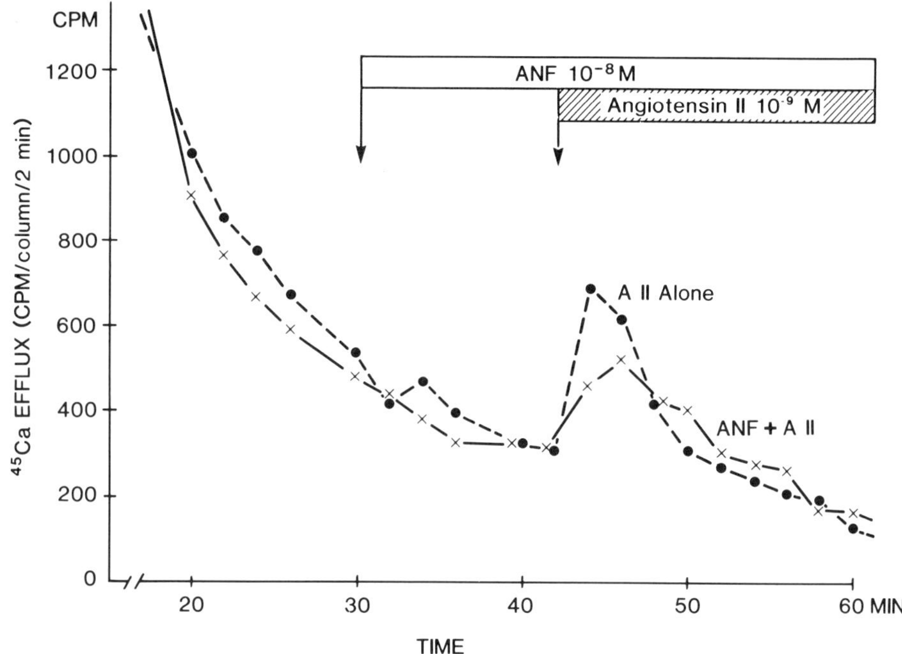

FIG. 12. Graph depicts efflux of ^{45}Ca from superfused adrenal zona glomerulosa cells prelabeled with ^{45}Ca. →, Start of superfusion. Length of bar, duration of superfusion. ●- - -●, ^{45}Ca efflux when only angiotensin II (AII) was superfused over adrenal cells. ×——×, ^{45}Ca efflux when ANF was superfused at first alone and then simultaneously with angiotensin II.

cyclase activity in adrenocortical membranes in a dose-dependent fashion. Matsuoka et al. (21) reported decreased cAMP production by rat adrenal glomerulosa cells in vitro in response to α-hANP. The effect on cAMP could explain in part the inhibition of ACTH activity but would not explain the inhibition of the action of angiotensin II. Furthermore, ANF can inhibit the stimulation of aldosterone by cAMP. Thus it has an additional action downstream from the generation of cAMP. Matsuoka et al. also reported stimulation of cGMP by α-hANP. The ANF is known to stimulate particulate guanylate cyclase but not the soluble enzyme in a variety of tissues. Whether this is the mechanism by which it inhibits aldosterone production is not clear. The threshold dose for stimulating cGMP production is usually higher than the dose to inhibit aldosterone. Also, the addition of derivatives of cGMP such as 8-bromo-cGMP to adrenal cells does not inhibit aldosterone production. Nevertheless the physiological significance of this effect of ANF on cGMP generation needs to be better understood. The membrane receptor for ANF and the membrane guanylate cyclase enzyme are closely associated.

Calcium: Intracellular and Extracellular

To understand how ANF can block all three stimuli, one would have to search for some factor that is an intermediate step in the stimulation of

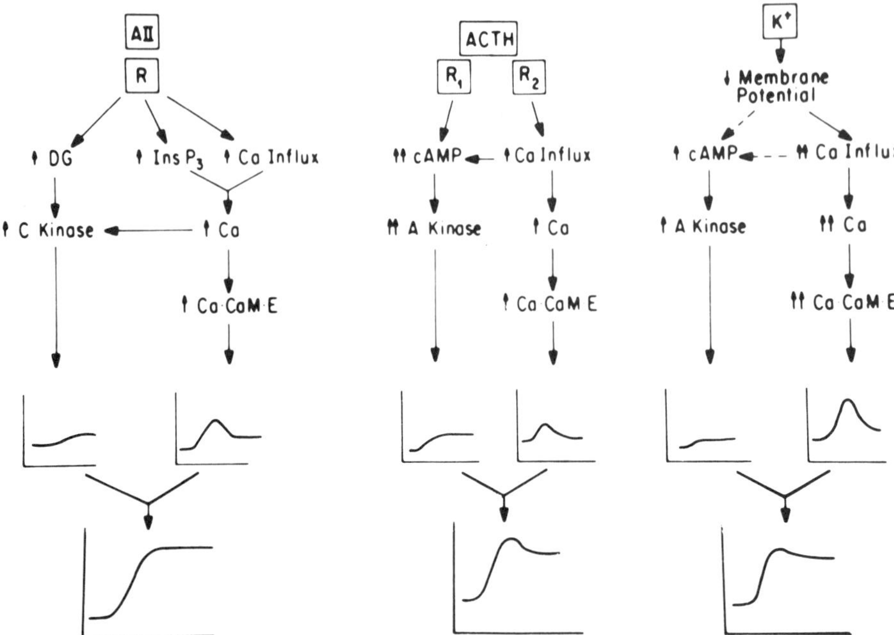

FIG. 13. Comparison of action of 3 agonists that regulate aldosterone production. AII, angiotensin II; R, receptor; DG, diacylglycerol; InsP₃, inositol triphosphate; Ca·CaM·E, calcium calmodulin–dependent enzymes. *Graphs*, aldosterone responses to different enzyme pathways; *bottom graphs*, synergistic responses. [From Kojima et al. (19).]

aldosterone production by the three stimuli. One such factor may be calcium. Angiotensin stimulates the turnover of phospholipids. After binding to its membrane receptor, angiotensin II activates phospholipase C, which in turn hydrolyzes phosphatidylinositol 4,5-biphosphate to diacylglycerol and inositol triphosphate. Inositol triphosphate mobilizes intracellular calcium from the endoplasmic reticulum to increase the concentration of free cytosolic calcium. The diacylglycerol, along with calcium, activates protein kinase C. Kojima et al. (18) blocked the intracellular mobilization of calcium with Dantrolene and inhibited the initial aldosterone response to angiotensin.

However, Goodfriend et al. (17) showed no effect of ANF on the increased turnover of phospholipids stimulated by angiotensin in bovine adrenal cells in vitro (23). We analyzed this system in another way. If glomerulosa cells are prelabeled with ^{45}Ca, the increase of free cytosolic calcium by angiotensin leads to a transient increase in the efflux of ^{45}Ca. Kojima et al. (18) have shown that Dantrolene blocked the efflux of ^{45}Ca stimulated by angiotensin and also the initial aldosterone response.

The results of a "typical" efflux experiment carried out by our group are shown in Figure 12. Rat adrenal glomerulosa cells were first prelabeled with ^{45}Ca and then placed on a Sephadex G-15 column and superfused with Krebs-Ringer-bicarbonate buffer. Rat atriopeptin, 1–28 ANP, or angiotensin II was added to the superfusate. Angiotensin alone transiently increases the calcium efflux from the prelabeled cells, as expected. When ANF is added before the addition of angiotensin and continued throughout the experiment, there is only a slight inhibition of ^{45}Ca efflux. However, the marked stimulation of aldosterone secretion by angiotensin to 368 pg/10^6 cells applied to the column per 2 min of collection of column effluent is almost completely inhibited by ANF (22 pg/10^6 cells per 2 min of collection). This result, therefore, appears to confirm the data of Goodfriend et al. (17) that ANF has little effect on phospholipid turnover and the initial mobilization of intracellular calcium. Nevertheless, calcium may be involved in other ways than through intracellular mobilization. It is known that a low-calcium medium or a calcium channel blocker such as verapamil attenuates the response of aldosterone production to all three stimuli (8, 12). More recently, Kojima et al. (19) emphasized the critical role of calcium influx in response to ACTH, angiotensin II, and potassium (Fig. 13). (The angiotensin II–hormone receptor interaction leads to two changes—an increase in plasma membrane calcium influx and the hydrolysis of phosphatidylinositol 4,5-biphosphate—which give rise to the two messengers, diacylglycerol and inositol triphosphate. Calcium calmodulin-dependent enzymes are activated and the cellular responses initiated. A rise in intracellular calcium along with the increase in diacylglycerol results in activation of protein kinase C. The protein kinase C remains in its calcium-sensitive state and regulates the sustained phase of cellular response. In the case of ACTH, interaction of hormone with the membrane leads to an increase in cAMP and in calcium influx. These activate cAMP-dependent protein kinase and calmodulin-dependent enzymes, which together result in the sustained aldosterone response. An increase in extracellular potassium concentration depolarizes the cell membrane and increases plasma membrane calcium influx and cAMP generation. These two messengers act similarly with ACTH, except there is a difference between the relative magnitude of the two messengers. The critical feature to all three stimuli is the cycling of calcium across the membrane, resulting in the activation of key enzymes that are required for this sustained response. We therefore suggest that ANF may act to reduce calcium influx across the plasma membrane and interfere with the activation of key enzymes needed for this sustained response to all three stimuli.

In summary, ANF has been demonstrated to inhibit aldosterone production by a direct adrenal action. This inhibition has been convincingly demonstrated for the three major stimuli of aldosterone in vitro. In vivo the evidence is less strong, although the data do support direct inhibition under most physiological conditions. The mechanism by which ANF affects the adrenal is not completely understood. A variety of actions have been demonstrated but no unifying first step has been identified to explain ANF's ability to inhibit all three stimuli.

Although early reports demonstrated an inhibitory effect on renin secretion, the more recent data are inconsistent. Renin may be decreased, increased, or unchanged by ANF. The result appears to depend on the experimental conditions.

REFERENCES

1. ANAND-SRIVASTAVA, M. B., J. GENEST, AND M. CANTIN. Inhibitory effect of atrial natriuretic factor on adenylate cyclase activity in adrenal cortical membranes. *FEBS Lett.* 181: 199–202, 1985.

2. ANDERSON, C., M. McCALLY, AND G. L. FANNELL. The effects of atrial stretch on aldosterone secretion. *Endocrinology* 64: 202–207, 1959.

3. ATARASHI, K., R. FRANCO-SAENZ, P. J. MULROW, R. M. SNAJDAR, AND J. P. RAPP. Inhibition of aldosterone production by atrial natriuretic factor. *J. Hypertens.* 2: 293–295, 1984.

4. ATARASHI, K., P. J. MULROW, AND R. FRANCO-SAENZ. Effect of atrial peptides on aldosterone production. *J. Clin. Invest.* 76: 1807–1811, 1985.

5. ATARASHI, K., P. J. MULROW, R. FRANCO-SAENZ, R. SNAJDAR, AND J. RAPP. Inhibition of aldosterone production by an atrial extract. *Science Wash. DC* 224: 992–994, 1984.

6. BURNETT, J. C., JR., J. P. GRANGER, AND T. J. OPGENORTH. Effects of synthetic atrial natriuretic factor on renal function and renin release. *Am. J. Physiol.* 247 (*Renal Fluid Electrolyte Physiol.* 16): F863–F866, 1984.

7. CAMPBELL, W. B., M. G. CURRIE, AND P. NEEDLEMAN. Inhibition of aldosterone biosynthesis by atriopeptins in rat adrenal cells. *Circ. Res.* 57: 113–118, 1985.

8. CAPPONI, A. M., P. D. LEW, L. JORNOT, AND M. B. VALLOTTON. Correlation between cytosolic free Ca^{2+} and aldosterone production in bovine adrenal glomerulosa cells. Evidence for a difference in the mode of action of angiotensin II and potassium. *J. Biol. Chem.* 259: 8863–8869, 1984.

9. CHARTIER, L., E. SCHIFFRIN, G. THIBAULT, AND R. GARCIA. Atrial natriuretic factor inhibits the stimulation of aldosterone secretion by angiotensin II, ACTH and potassium in vitro and angiotensin II-induced steroidogenesis in vivo. *Endocrinology* 115: 2026–2028, 1984.

10. DE LÉAN, A., K. RACZ, J. GUTKOWSKA, T.-T. NGUYEN, M. CANTIN, AND J. GENEST. Specific receptor-mediated inhibition by synthetic atrial natriuretic factor of hormone-stimulated steroidogenesis in cultured bovine adrenal cells. *Endocrinology* 115: 1636–1638, 1984.

11. DENTON, D. A., J. R. BLAIR-WEST, J. P. COGHLAN, B. A. SCOGGINS, AND R. D. WRIGHT. Gustatory-alimentary reflex inhibition of aldosterone hypersecretion by the autotransplanted adrenal gland of sodium deficient sheep. *Acta Endocrinol.* 84: 119–132, 1977.

12. FAKUNDING, J. L., AND K. J. CATT. Dependence of aldosterone stimulation in adrenal glomerulosa cells on calcium uptake: effects of lanthanum and verapamil. *Endocrinology* 107: 1345–1353, 1980.

13. FREEMAN, R. H., J. O. DAVIS, AND R. C. VARI. Renal response to atrial natriuretic factor in conscious dogs with caval constriction. *Am. J. Physiol.* 248 (*Regulatory Integrative Comp. Physiol.* 17): R495–R500, 1985.

14. GANN, D. S., AND R. H. TRAVIS. Mechanisms of hemodynamic control of secretion of aldosterone in the dog. *Am. J. Physiol.* 207: 1095–1101, 1964.

15. GARCIA, R., J. GUTKOWSKA, J. GENEST, M. CANTIN, AND G. THIBAULT. Reduction of blood pressure and increased diuresis and natriuresis during chronic infusion of atrial natriuretic factor (ANF Arg 101-Tyr 126) in conscious one-kidney, one-clip hypertensive rats. *Proc. Soc. Exp. Biol. Med.* 179: 539–545, 1985.

16. GARCIA, R., G. THIBAULT, J. GUTKOWSKA, P. HAMET, M. CANTIN, AND J. GENEST. Effect of chronic infusion of synthetic atrial natriuretic factor (ANF 8-33) in conscious two-kidney, one-clip hypertensive rats. *Proc. Soc. Exp. Biol. Med.* 178: 155–159, 1985.

17. GOODFRIEND, T. L., M. E. ELLIOTT, AND S. A. ATLAS. Actions of synthetic atrial natriuretic factor on bovine adrenal glomerulosa. *Life Sci.* 35: 1675–1682, 1984.

18. KOJIMA, I., K. KOJIMA, AND H. RASMUSSEN. Effects of ANG II and K^+ on Ca efflux and aldosterone production in adrenal glomerulosa cells. *Am. J. Physiol.* 248 (*Endocrinol. Metab.* 11): E36–E43, 1985.

19. KOJIMA, I., K. KOJIMA, AND H. RASMUSSEN. Role of calcium and cAMP in the action of adrenocorticotropin on aldosterone secretion. *J. Biol. Chem.* 260: 4248–4256, 1985.

20. MAACK, T., D. N. MARION, M. J. CAMARGO, H. D. KLEINERT, J. H. LARAGH, E. D. VAUGHAN, JR., AND S. A. ATLAS. Effects of auriculin (atrial natriuretic factor) on blood pressure, renal function, and the renin-aldosterone system in dogs. *Am. J. Med.* 77: 1069–1075, 1984.

21. MATSUOKA, H., M. ISHII, T. SUGIMOTO, Y. HIRATA, T. SUGIMOTO, K. KANGAWA, AND H. MATSUO. Inhibition of aldosterone production by α-human atrial natriuretic polypeptide is associated with an increase in cGMP production. *Biochem. Biophys. Res. Commun.* 127: 1052–1056, 1985.

22. MILLS, I. H., A. CASPER, AND F. C. BARTTER. On the role of the vagus in the control of aldosterone secretion. *Science Wash. DC* 128: 1140–1141, 1958.
23. OBANA, K., M. NARUSE, K. NARUSE, H. SAKURAI, H. DEMURA, T. INAGAMI, AND K. SHIZUME. Synthetic rat atrial natriuretic factor inhibits in vitro and in vivo renin secretion in rats. *Endocrinology* 117: 1282–1284, 1985.
24. RICHARDS, A. M., M. G. NICHOLLS, E. A. ESPINER, H. IKRAM, T. G. YANDLE, S. L. JOYCE, AND M. M. CULLENS. Effects of α-human atrial natriuretic peptide in essential hypertension. *Hypertension Dallas* 7: 812–817, 1985.
25. SEYMOUR, A. A., E. H. BLAINE, E. K. MAZACK, S. G. SMITH, I. I. STABILITO, A. B. HALEY, M. A. NAPIER, M. A. WHINNERY, AND R. F. NUTT. Renal and systemic effects of synthetic atrial natriuretic factor. *Life Sci.* 36: 33–34, 1985.
26. TAKAGI, M., R. FRANCO-SAENZ, AND P. J. MULROW. Effect of atrial natriuretic factor on the plasma aldosterone response to potassium infusion in rats—in vivo study. *Life Sci.* 39: 359–364, 1986.
27. TAKAGI, M., M. TAKAGI, R. FRANCO-SAENZ, AND P. J. MULROW. Synthetic rat natriuretic factor does not inhibit in vitro and in vivo renin secretion in rats (abstr.). *Clin. Res.* 34: 611A, 1986.
28. TIKKANEN, I., K. METSÄRINNE, F. FYHRQUIST, AND R. LEIDENIUS. Plasma atrial natriuretic peptide in cardiac disease and during infusion in healthy volunteers. *Lancet* 2: 66–69, 1985.
29. VOLPE, M., G. ODELL, H. D. KLEINERT, F. MÜLLER, M. J. CAMARGO, J. H. LARAGH, T. MAACK, E. D. VAUGHAN, JR., AND S. ATLAS. Effect of atrial natriuretic factor on blood pressure, renin, and aldosterone in Goldblatt hypertension. *Hypertension Dallas* 7: 143–148, 1985.
30. WALDHAUSEL, W., H. VIERHAPPER, AND P. NOWOTNY. Prolonged administration of human atrial natriuretic peptide in healthy men: evanescent effects of diuresis and natriuresis. *J. Clin. Endocrinol. Metab.* 62: 956–959, 1986.
31. WEIDMANN, P., L. HASLER, P. GNADINGER, R. E. LANG, D. E. UEHLINGER, S. SHAW, W. RASCHER, AND F. C. REUBI. Blood levels and renal effects of atrial natriuretic peptide in normal man. *J. Clin. Invest.* 77: 734–742, 1986.
32. WEIDMANN, P., B. HELLMUELLER, D. E. UEHLINGER, R. E. LANG, M. P. GNAEDINGER, L. HASLER, S. SHAW, AND C. BACHMANN. Plasma levels and cardiovascular, endocrine, and excretory effects of atrial natriuretic peptide during different sodium intakes in man. *J. Clin. Endocrinol. Metab.* 62: 1027–1036, 1986.

10

Atrial Natriuretic Factor in Animal Models for Hypertension

JOHN P. RAPP

Departments of Medicine and Pathology, Medical College of Ohio, Toledo, Ohio

Spontaneously Hypertensive Rats
Dahl Rats
Renal Hypertension
Other Animal Models of Hypertension
Conclusion

THE DISCOVERY OF ATRIAL NATRIURETIC FACTOR (ANF) has generated great interest in the field of hypertension. The important questions with regard to hypertension are *1)* does a deficiency in ANF secretion or ANF responsiveness function in the pathogenesis of hypertension and *2)* does ANF lower blood pressure in the hypertensive state. These questions are reviewed in animal models for hypertension.

SPONTANEOUSLY HYPERTENSIVE RATS

Comparison of the atrial content of ANF in spontaneously hypertensive rats (SHR) and normotensive control Wistar-Kyoto rats (WKY) by bioassay indicated lower ANF per atrium in SHR (24). By radioimmunoassay it was found that the concentration of ANF per unit weight of atrium was similar in SHR and WKY at weaning. As hypertension developed with age, ANF in the left atrium of the SHR decreased but that in the right atrium was unchanged (6, 14). In another report (4) ANF was measured by radioimmunoassay but the data were expressed per gram of total heart. In this case also, cardiac ANF in SHR and WKY was comparable at a young age and was less in SHR than in WKY in adults when SHR had become hypertensive. Although SHR in this report had mild cardiac hypertrophy, the total heart content of ANF still appeared lower in adult SHR than WKY. No qualitative differences in the ANF immunoreactive molecules were detected by gel-filtration chromatography or by reverse-phase high-pressure liquid chromatography (HPLC) (4, 6, 14).

Plasma ANF in SHR has been found to be lower than in WKY by Higa et al. (4), but the plasma levels reported by these authors are clearly much too high compared with numerous measurements on rat plasma in the literature. These data are probably invalid because they were obtained on blood collected by decapitation (which contaminates the blood with tissue proteases), without the use of protease inhibitors and without an extraction procedure that would also minimize proteolysis. The data of Imada et al. (6) and Morii et al. (14) are more likely to be correct; i.e., plasma ANF is similar in young SHR and WKY, but as the rats age and SHR become hypertensive, plasma ANF increases severalfold in SHR but not in WKY.

Because ANF is in the nervous system and may function as a neuropeptide transmitter, or modulator, it has been measured in the brain of SHR. In the hypothalamus and pons, ANF was higher in SHR than WKY at 8 wk of age and after but not at weaning (6).

The influence of infused atrial peptide on blood pressure has been studied in SHR because these peptides are known to relax vascular smooth muscle. Although many different doses and infusion protocols have been used, there is a consensus that ANF reduces blood pressure in chronic infusions and the effect on blood pressure is greater in SHR than WKY (3, 12, 15, 17, 19). It is typical for a hypotensive agent to reduce blood pressure more in a hypertensive than in a normotensive animal, but the reason for this is obscure.

Although one would expect the decreased blood pressure in SHR in response to ANF to be due to its vasodilatory properties, this is not necessarily the case. Cardiac output was reduced by ANF (10, 16, 17) and total peripheral resistance was increased (10). The increased vascular resistance observed has been interpreted as a neurally mediated reflex response in an attempt to maintain blood pressure in the face of decreased cardiac output (10). When SHR were sympathectomized with 6-hydroxydopamine, instead of causing increased vascular resistance, ANF infusion was associated with a decrease in vascular resistance (11). The mechanism by which ANF decreases cardiac output is not established, but ANF has been reported to decrease coronary blood flow (26).

The diuretic and natriuretic responses to ANF have been reported to be decreased in SHR (12) or increased in SHR (7, 9, 15) relative to WKY. Urinary cGMP, which is known to be increased by ANF, increased much less in SHR than WKY (12), suggesting renal hyporesponsiveness in the hypertensive strain. Pang et al. (15), however, reported that ANF caused similar changes in cGMP in SHR and WKY. Smith et al. (19) report that SHR do not show renal vasodilation in response to ANF. In contrast, Koike et al. (8) reported that ANF selectively increases blood flow in SHR. Neither Smith et al. nor Koike et al. included studies on a control strain; thus the data are uninterpretable in genetic terms.

DAHL RATS

Two strains of rats were selectively bred by Dahl: one is sensitive (S) to the hypertensive effect of a high-salt diet; the other is resistant (R) to salt-induced hypertension. Because of the involvement of sodium in the development of hypertension in S rats, the study of ANF in these strains is especially germane.

It has been shown by bioassay that Dahl S rats have a higher concentration of ANF in their atria than Dahl R rats (5, 22). These bioassay findings have been confirmed by radioimmunoassay (20, 21). It was also found that between 1 and 15 days of age ANF heart content was equal in S and R rats. The strains diverge at 30 days of age, with S rats having more ANF in atria than R rats, a difference that persists through 6 mo of age. Increasing or decreasing salt in the diet did not remove the difference in ANF atrial concentration in the S and R rats (20, 22). In another report no difference in S and R atrial ANF was found by radioimmunoassay (25), but this study has two major drawbacks: it used few rats and it used outbred Dahl rats instead of the more highly salt-sensitive, recently developed inbred strains of Dahl rats. No qualitative differences in the various atrial natriuretic polypeptides were found between S and R rats by reverse-phase HPLC or gel-filtration chromatography (20, 25).

Plasma ANF is not different in strains of Dahl rats in situations where the S and R rats have similar blood pressures (young rats or low-salt diet). When blood pressure of S and R rats is markedly different, (high-salt diet or 6-mo-old rats), S rats have plasma ANF concentrations severalfold higher than R rats (23, 25). Table 1 gives examples of plasma ANF values (21). No qualitative difference in plasma ANF as evaluated by reverse-phase HPLC was found (23, 25).

Renal natriuretic and diuretic responses of S rats are reduced compared with R rats when the rats are young (5, 22). As animals age and S rats develop hypertension, the situation is reversed; i.e., S rats are now hyperresponsive and excrete more salt and water to a given challenge with ANF (22). This reversal is interpreted to result from the effects of high blood pressure directly on renal function or to be the result of renal (glomerular) lesions, which are always present in hypertensive S rats.

RENAL HYPERTENSION

In both the one-kidney, one clip and two-kidney, one clip models of renal hypertension in the rat, ANF infusion lowers systolic blood pressure 30–70 mmHg (1, 2, 18). The effect of ANF in similarly treated normotensive controls

TABLE 1. *Blood pressure and immunoreactive ANF in plasma of Dahl R and S rats*

	R		S		P		
	Low salt	High salt	Low salt	High salt	Strain	Diet	Inter-action
Blood pressure, mmHg	96.6 ± 2.5* (10)	99.8 ± 3.4 (10)	120.1 ± 3.8 (10)	175 ± 6.8 (10)	<0.001	<0.001	<0.001
Plasma ANF, pg/ml	237 ± 65.2 (10)	270 ± 89.1 (10)	209 ± 26.7 (10)	897 ± 294.4 (9)	0.012	0.004	0.013

Dahl R rats, resistant to salt-induced hypertension; Dahl S rats, sensitive to salt-induced hypertension. Rats were fed low-salt (0.4% NaCl) or high-salt (80% NaCl) diet for 21 days, starting at 4 wk of age. Number of rats in parentheses. Plasma ANF is in picograms of atriopeptin III equivalents per milliliter. *P* determined from a 2 × 2 factorial analysis of variance; plasma ANF was analyzed with a logarithmic transformation to equalize variances among groups. * Mean ± SE.

was much less pronounced; a decrease ranging from 0 to 20 mmHg was observed. The effects of ANF on water and sodium excretion in renal hypertension were variable. In some cases increased natriuresis and diuresis were present when blood pressure was reduced (1); in other cases they were not (2, 18). Whether ANF decreased blood pressure through effects on blood volume is unclear.

OTHER ANIMAL MODELS OF HYPERTENSION

Infusion of ANF has been shown to reduce high blood pressure caused by deoxycorticosterone plus saline to drink (18) or caused by norepinephrine (27).

McKenzie et al. (13) studied ANF in pulmonary hypertension induced by exposures to chronic hypobaric hypoxia. Plasma ANF went up twofold. Right atrial ANF concentration decreased and left atrial ANF concentraton increased, suggesting that the right atrium was the source of the increased plasma ANF. This is the expected result if atrial stretch is the stimulus for release of ANF.

CONCLUSION

One would anticipate that if ANF has a role in the development of hypertension, either secretion of ANF or responses to ANF would be reduced. In genetically hypertensive rats, plasma ANF is increased, not decreased, when the rats develop hypertension; this has been interpreted as a result of hypertension, not as a cause of hypertension. Renal natriuretic and diuretic responses to ANF in various animal models have usually increased, not decreased, as would be expected if end-organ hyporesponsiveness were a cause of hypertension. An important exception is the Dahl S rat, in which the kidneys were hyporesponsive to ANF, but only in young rats prior to the development of hypertension. As hypertension develops, renal responses to ANF are altered. This points up the necessity for studying developmental patterns when working with genetically hypertensive rats.

There is an interesting contrast between SHR and Dahl S rats with regard to the atrial content of ANF. Dahl S rats appear to have higher atrial ANF relative to their appropriate control strain, whereas SHR appear to have lower atrial ANF relative to their appropriate control strain. In neither SHR nor S rats is there any evidence for a qualitative difference in the ANF molecule. Since both strains increase plasma ANF dramatically as they become hypertensive, the meaning of the tissue concentration differences is obscure.

In all hypertensive animal models tested, ANF markedly decreased blood pressure. The mechanism by which it does this appears somewhat surprisingly to be through decreases in cardiac output, rather than through effects on volume regulation or vasodilation. Certainly this point will receive further investigation.

This work was supported by National Institutes of Health Grants HL-20176 and HL-34394.

REFERENCES

1. GARCIA, R., J. GUTKOWSKA, J. GENEST, M. CANTIN, G. THIBAULT. Reduction of blood pressure and increased diuresis and natriuresis during chronic infusion of atrial natriuretic factor (ANF Arg 101-Tyr 126) in conscious one-kidney, one-clip hypertensive rats. *Proc. Soc. Exp. Biol. Med.* 179: 539–545, 1985.
2. GARCIA, R., G. THIBAULT, J. GUTKOWSKA, P. HAMET, M. CANTIN, AND J. GENEST. Effect of chronic infusion of synthetic atrial natriuretic factor (ANF 8-33) in conscious two-kidney, one-clip hypertensive rats. *Proc. Soc. Exp. Biol. Med.* 178: 155–159, 1985.
3. GARCIA, R., G. THIBAULT, J. GUTKOWSKA, K. HORKÝ, P. HAMET, M. CANTIN, AND J. GENEST. Chronic infusion of low doses of atrial natriuretic factor (ANF Arg 101-Tyr 126) reduces blood pressure in conscious SHR without apparent changes in sodium excretion. *Proc. Soc. Exp. Biol. Med.* 179: 396–401, 1985.
4. HIGA, T., K. KITAMURA, A. MIGATA, K. KANGAWA, H. MATSUO, AND K. TANAKA. Cardiac content and plasma concentration of atrial natriuretic polypeptide (ANP) in spontaneously hypertensive rats (SHR). *Jpn. Circ. J.* 49: 973–979, 1985.
5. HIRATA, Y., M. GANGULI, L. TOBIAN, AND J. IWAI. Dahl S rats have increased natriuretic factor in atria but are markedly hyporesponsive to it. *Hypertension Dallas* 6, Suppl. I: I148–I155, 1984.
6. IMADA, T., R. TAKAYANAGI, AND T. INAGAMI. Changes in the content of atrial natriuretic factor with the progression of hypertension in spontaneously hypertensive rats. *Biochem. Biophys. Res. Commun.* 133: 759–765, 1985.
7. KIHARA, M., K. NAKAYAMA, K. NAKAO, A. SUGAWARA, N. MORII, M. SAKAMOTO, M. SUDA, M. SHIMOKURA, Y. KISO, H. IMURA, AND Y. YAMORI. Accelerated natriuresis induced by synthetic atrial natriuretic polypeptide in spontaneously hypertensive rats. *Clin. Exp. Hypertens. Part A Theory Pract.* 7: 539–551, 1985.
8. KOIKE, H., T. SADA, M. MIYAMOTO, K. OIZUMI, M. SUGIYAMA, AND T. INAGAMI. Atrial natriuretic factor selectively increases renal blood flow in conscious spontaneously hypertensive rats. *Eur. J. Pharmacol.* 104: 391–392, 1984.
9. KONDO, K., O. KIDA, K. KANGAWA, H. MATSUO, AND K. TANAKA. Enhanced natriuretic and hypotensive responsiveness to α-human atrial natriuretic polypeptide (α-h ANP) in SHR. *Clin. Exp. Hypertens. Part A Theory Pract.* 7: 1097–1107, 1985.
10. LAPPE, R. W., J. F. M. SMITS, J. A. TODT, J. J. M. DEBETS, AND R. L. WENDT. Failure of atriopeptin II to cause arterial vasodilation in the conscious rat. *Circ. Res.* 56: 606–612, 1985.
11. LAPPE, R. W., J. A. TODT, AND R. L. WENDT. Mechanism of action of vasoconstrictor responses to atriopeptin II in conscious SHR. *Am. J. Physiol.* 249 (*Regulatory Integrative Comp. Physiol.* 18): R781–R786, 1985.
12. MARSH, A., A. A. SEYMOUR, A. B. HALEY, M. A. WHINNERY, M. A. NAPIER, R. F. NUTT, AND E. H. BLAINE. Renal and blood pressure responses to synthetic atrial natriuretic factor in spontaneously hypertensive rats. *Hypertension Dallas* 7: 386–391, 1985.
13. MCKENZIE, J. C., I. TANAKA, T. INAGAMI, K. S. MISONO, AND R. M. KLEIN. Alterations in atrial and plasma atrial natriuretic factor (ANF) content during development of hypoxia-induced pulmonary hypertension in the rat. *Proc. Soc. Exp. Biol. Med.* 181: 459–463, 1986.
14. MORII, N., K. NAKAO, M. KIHARA, A. SUGANARA, M. SAKAMOTO, Y. YAMORI, AND H. IMURA. Decreased content in left atrium and increased plasma concentration of atrial natriuretic polypeptide in spontaneously hypertensive rats (SHR) and stroke-prone SHR. *Biochim. Biophys. Acta* 135: 74–81, 1986.
15. PANG, S. C., M. HOANG, J. TREMPLAY, M. CANTIN, R. GARCIA, J. GENEST, AND P. HAMET. Effect of natural and synthetic atrial natriuretic factor on arterial blood pressure, natriuresis and cyclic GMP excretion in spontaneously hypertensive rats. *Clin. Sci. Lond.* 69: 721–726, 1985.
16. PEGRAM, B. L., M. B. KARDON, N. C. TRIPPODO, F. E. COLE, AND A. A. MACPHEE. Atrial extract: hemodynamics in Wistar-Kyoto and spontaneously hypertensive rats. *Am. J. Physiol.* 249 (*Heart Circ. Physiol.* 18): H265–H271, 1985.
17. SASAKI, A., O. KIDA, K. KANGAWA, H. MATSUO, AND K. TANAKA. Cardiosuppressive effect of α-human atrial natriuretic polypeptide (α-hANP) in spontaneously hypertensive rats. *Eur. J. Pharmacol.* 115: 321–324, 1985.
18. SEYMOUR, A. A., E. A. MARSH, E. K. MAZACK, I. I. STABILITO, AND E. H. BLAINE. Synthetic atrial natriuretic factor in conscious normotensive and hypertensive rats. *Hypertension Dallas* 7, Suppl. I: I35–I42, 1985.

19. SMITH, J. F. M., H. VAN ESSEN, H. A. J. STRUYKER-BOUDIER, AND R. W. LAPPE. Lack of renal vasodilation during intrarenal infusion of synthetic atriopeptin II in conscious intact SHR. *Life Sci.* 38: 81–87, 1986.

20. SNAJDAR, R. M., H. DENE, AND J. P. RAPP. Partial characterization of atrial natriuretic polypeptide in the hearts of Dahl salt-sensitive and salt-resistant rats. *Endocrinology.* In press.

21. SNAJDAR, R. M., H. DENE, AND J. P. RAPP. Atrial natriuretic factor in inbred Dahl salt-sensitive and salt-resistant rats. *J. Hypertens.* In press.

22. SNAJDAR, R. M., AND J. P. RAPP. Atrial natriuretic factor in Dahl rats. Atrial content and renal and aortic responses. *Hypertension Dallas* 7: 775–782, 1985.

23. SNAJDAR, R. M., AND J. P. RAPP. Elevated atrial natriuretic polypeptide in plasma of hypertensive Dahl salt-sensitive rats. *Biochem. Biophys. Res. Commun.* 137: 876–883, 1986.

24. SONNENBERG, H., S. MILOJEVIC, C. K. CHONG, AND A. T. VERESS. Atrial natriuretic factor: reduced cardiac content in spontaneously hypertensive rats. *Hypertension Dallas* 5: 672–675, 1983.

25. TANAKA, I., AND T. INAGAMI. Increased concentration of plasma immunoreactive atrial natriuretic factor in Dahl salt-sensitive rats with sodium chloride-induced hypertension. *J. Hypertens.* 4: 109–112, 1986.

26. WANGLER, R. D., B. A. BREUHAUS, H. O. OTERO, D. A. HASTINGS, M. D. HOLZMAN, H. H. SANEII, H. V. SPARKS, AND J. E. CHIMOSKEY. Coronary vasoconstrictor effects of atriopeptin II. *Science Wash. DC* 230: 558–561, 1985.

27. YASUJIMA, M., K. ABE, M. KOHZUKI, M. TANNO, Y. KASAI, M. SATO, K. OMATA, K. KUDO, T. TSUNODA, K. TAKEUCHI, K. YOSHINGA, AND T. INAGAMI. Atrial natriuretic factor inhibits the hypertension induced by chronic infusion of norepinephrine in conscious rats. *Circ. Res.* 57: 470–474, 1985.

11

Effect of Human Atrial Natriuretic Peptide in Normal and Hypertensive Humans

ERIC A. ESPINER, M. GARY NICHOLLS, A. MARK RICHARDS, ROSS C. CUNEO, TIM G. YANDLE, AND HAMID IKRAM

Departments of Endocrinology and Cardiology, The Princess Margaret Hospital, Christchurch, New Zealand

Effects of Intravenous Bolus of α-Human Atrial Natriuretic Peptide (ANP) Constant Infusions of α-Human ANP and Effect of Sodium Intake on Response

AT LEAST THREE CHEMICALLY RELATED POLYPEPTIDES with natriuretic and vasorelaxant effects in experimental animals have been isolated from human atrial tissue (5). Although the precise identity of the circulating forms in human plasma is still unknown, there is good evidence that the 28–amino acid peptide, α-human atrial natriuretic peptide (α-hANP), or a closely similar peptide is a major component of the circulating immunoreactivity in humans (18) and is subject to physiological regulation (3). Furthermore, elevated levels occur in a wide variety of clinical disorders associated with hypervolemia (3). These findings, which are consistent with other reports in mammals (8, 15), suggest that α-hANP has a hormonal function that could be important in extracellular fluid volume homeostasis. Crucial to this view is the demonstration of biological activity of α-hANP in the species of origin. Accordingly we have used intravenous bolus injections and constant infusions of α-hANP to study the renal, endocrine, and hemodynamic effects in normal and hypertensive humans. The effect of sodium intake on these responses has also been studied.

EFFECTS OF INTRAVENOUS BOLUS OF α-HUMAN ANP

Given as an intravenous bolus (over 60 s) to six normotensive volunteers equilibrated on a daily sodium intake of 120 mmol, 100 μg of α-hANP produced a prompt and major increase in sodium, calcium, magnesium, phosphorus, and urine volume when compared with a placebo injection given on another day (14). As shown in Figure 1, sodium excretion increased fourfold when there were no significant changes in potassium or creatinine excretion. Compared to normotensives, hypertensive subjects studied under the same conditions showed a greater response of urine volume, sodium, calcium, and magnesium excretion (13). There was a sixfold increase in sodium output in the initial 30 min after α-hANP injection, and the cumulative excretion of sodium in

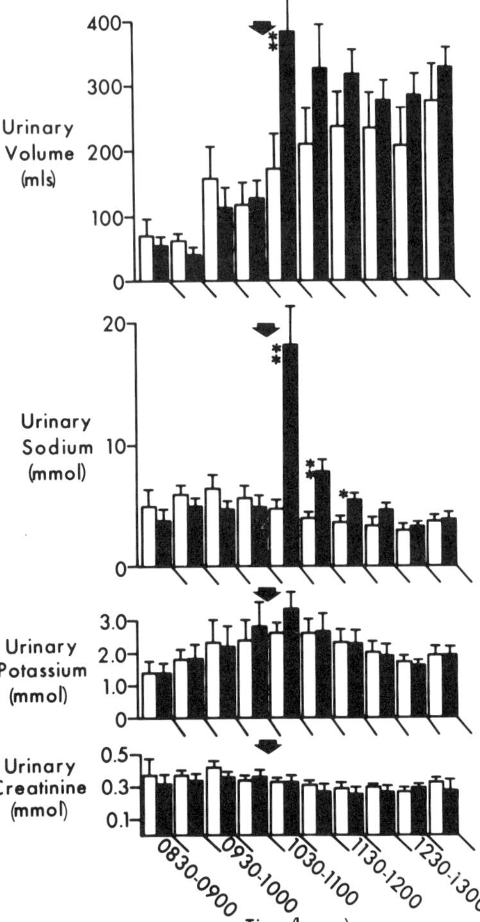

FIG. 1. Urinary volume, sodium, potassium, and creatinine excretion (mean ± SE) before and after administration (*arrow*) of placebo (*open columns*) or 100 µg α-human atrial natriuretic peptide (α-hANP) (*filled columns*) to 6 normotensive volunteers. *$P < 0.05$ for differences between ANP and placebo; **$P < 0.01$. [From Richards et al. (14).]

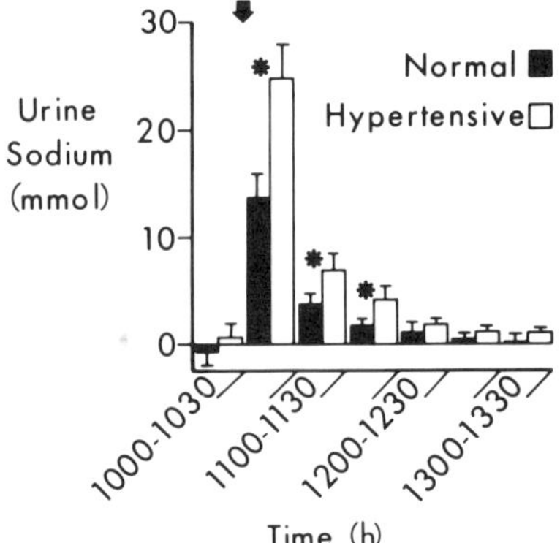

FIG. 2. Urinary sodium excretion (mean ± SE) in excess of that on the time-matched placebo day calculated from 30-min collection periods in 6 hypertensives (*open columns*) and 6 normotensive volunteers (*filled columns*) before and after injection (*arrow*) of 100 µg α-hANP. *$P < 0.05$. [From Richards et al. (13), by permission of the American Heart Association, Inc.]

hypertensive subjects exceeded that in normotensive subjects (Fig. 2). This exaggerated urinary response could not be explained by differences in the plasma immunoreactive ANP (IR-ANP) concentration achieved after injection, since the mean level 15-min postinjection in hypertensives (203 ± 4 pM) was lower than that of normotensives (342 ± 20 pM), in keeping with the higher body weight of the hypertensive subjects (mean 81 kg vs. 71 kg in normotensives). The amount of sodium excreted in the 30 min postinjection of α-hANP correlated positively with the level of intra-arterial pressure measured continuously (10) 30 min prior to the injection (Fig. 3). This positive correlation of urine sodium excretion with arterial pressure was also present within each of the two groups. While atrial peptides appear to be less natriuretic when blood pressure falls acutely (17), the effect of a sustained elevation in arterial pressure on the renal response to ANP is still controversial (6, 12). Our findings in a small group of volunteers agree with some experimental findings (11, 17) that show enhanced natriuresis to ANP in hypertensive animals.

The injection of 100 μg α-hANP in normotensive subjects produced an immediate small but consistent fall in arterial pressure and a significant increase in heart rate, as measured by the Oxford technique of continuous pressure and heart-rate recording (10). Figure 4 shows the response to intravenous α-hANP and placebo injections in one normal subject. These changes in blood pressure and heart rate, compared with control observations, were sustained for up to two hours after injection of α-hANP. However, in hypertensives, while the sustained increase in heart rate was observed, mean arterial pressure fell only briefly and had returned to control levels 10 min after α-hANP (Fig. 5). Associated with these hemodynamic effects were transient increases in plasma norepinephrine and a later fall in plasma epinephrine concentration in hypertensive subjects. Other hormones including plasma renin activity (PRA), plasma arginine vasopressin, and cortisol did not change significantly in either the normal or hypertensive group. However, plasma aldosterone tended to fall after α-hANP injection in normal subjects and plasma aldosterone was significantly reduced 30–40 min after α-hANP injection in hypertensives (13). No ill effects were reported by subjects receiving α-hANP. However, 7 of 12 subjects given an intravenous bolus of 100 μg noted

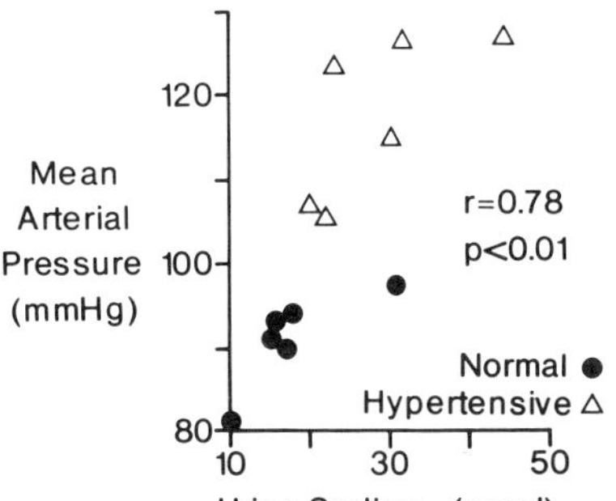

FIG. 3. Relation between mean intra-arterial pressure measured continuously for 30 min (from 1000 to 1030) and sodium excretion (from 1030 to 1100) immediately after 100 μg α-hANP. [From Richards et al. (13), by permission of the American Heart Association, Inc.]

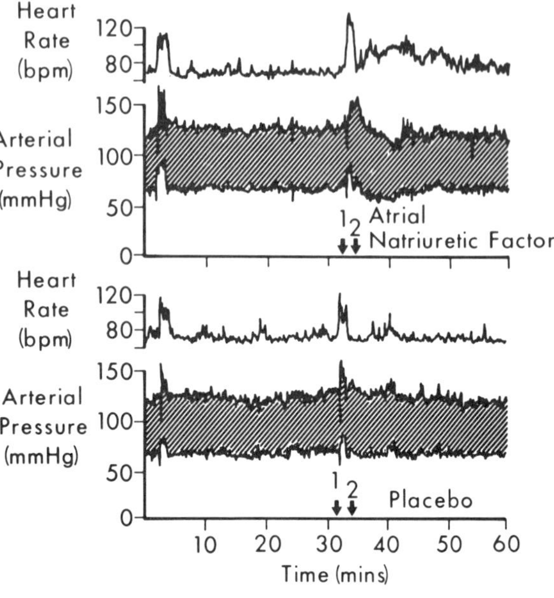

FIG. 4. Heart rate and intra-arterial pressure recorded continuously for 60 min in one normotensive volunteer before and after injection (*arrow 2*) of α-hANP (*top panel*) and placebo (*bottom panel*). *Arrow 1*, change from sitting to standing posture to pass urine. Rise in heart rate and fall in blood pressure observed after α-hANP injection do not occur on the control day.

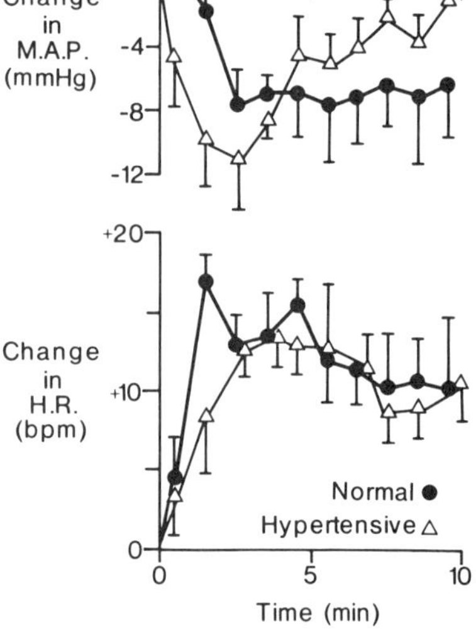

FIG. 5. Changes in heart rate (HR) and mean intra-arterial pressure (MAP) after injection of 100 μg α-hANP in 6 normal and 6 hypertensive subjects. Changes are based on mean continuous recordings for 30 min (from 1000 to 1030) before injection. Data are means ± SE.

a transient facial-flushing sensation within minutes after the injection, whereas none complained of this after the placebo injection.

These results confirm the biological activity of α-hANP in humans and suggest that the hormone has a greater natriuretic activity in subjects with hypertension. However, in view of the rapid metabolism of α-hANP, which has a plasma half-life of ~3 min in humans (19), studies that use bolus injections were of limited value in clarifying the hormone's physiological action. For these reasons, constant intravenous infusions of α-hANP were

used to relate physiological actions to steady-state plasma concentrations of
α-hANP.

CONSTANT INFUSIONS OF α-HUMAN ANP AND EFFECT OF SODIUM INTAKE ON RESPONSE

When 200 μg α-hANP were given as a constant intravenous infusion over
60 min to six normotensive male volunteers equilibrated on a daily sodium
intake of 200 mmol, sodium excretion increased more than threefold (Fig. 6)
and comparable and significant increases in calcium and magnesium excretion
also occurred (2a). Most of these indices had returned to control-day levels in
the second 30-min collection period after cessation of the infusion. A small,
transient increase in potassium excretion was not sustained and failed to
achieve statistical significance when compared with control-day observations.
There was no significant change in urine creatinine excretion or endogenous
creatinine clearance during α-hANP infusions. These changes in electrolyte
excretion and the increase in urine volume occurred at mean steady-state
venous plasma concentrations of IR-ANP of 320 pM. High-performance liquid
chromatography analysis of extracts of plasma taken at 45 and 60 min after
commencing an α-hANP infusion confirmed that α-hANP was the major
contributor to IR-ANP measured in plasma. Data from experimental animals
have shown a dose-dependent natriuresis over the range 6.25–100 pmol·kg^{-1}·
min^{-1} (16). Our results in humans with infusion rates approximating 15 pmol·
kg^{-1}·min^{-1} are similar to those of Maack et al. (9) in anesthetized dogs
receiving 26–30 pmol·kg^{-1}·min^{-1}. Thus it appears that the natriuretic re-

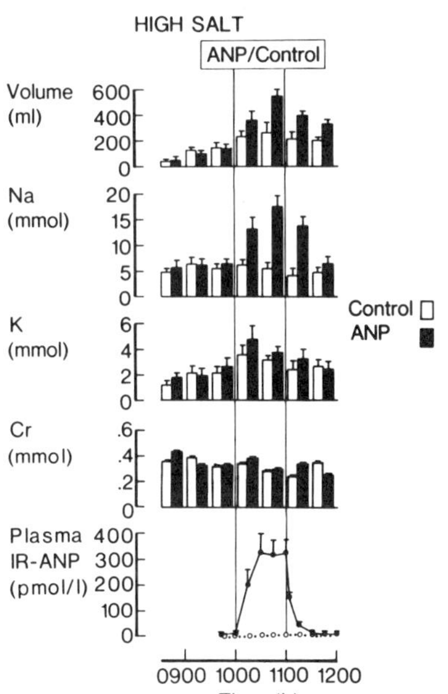

FIG. 6. Urinary volume, sodium, potassium, and
creatinine excretion before, during, and after control
(*open columns*) and α-hANP (*filled columns*) infusions
in 6 normal subjects equilibrated on a 200 mmol
sodium intake. Plasma levels of immunoreactive ANP
(IR-ANP) are also shown for ANP infusion (*filled
circles*) and control (*open circles*) days. Results are
means ± SE.

sponse to α-hANP in humans is at least as sensitive as that observed in some animals. To determine whether sodium intake affects the renal response, we also studied the response of the same six normotensive subjects given an identical infusion of α-hANP (200 μg over 60 min) when equilibrated on a daily sodium intake of 10 mmol. Steady-state plasma IR-ANP levels achieved during infusions were the same as those on the 200-mmol diet, indicating that the metabolic clearance rate of α-hANP in humans is unaffected by major changes in sodium intake. As shown in Figure 7, peak natriuresis was markedly reduced (~10% of that observed on the high-salt diet), although the response in urine volume and magnesium excretion was similar on the two different diets. Others studying dogs (4) have observed a diminished natriuretic response to atrial peptides in the setting of enhanced renal tubular avidity for sodium. Our results in humans suggest that both preexisting systemic pressure and sodium status are important determinants of the natriuretic response to α-hANP.

In contrast to the effect of a 100-μg bolus of α-hANP, we found no significant hypotensive effect of α-hANP infusions given to normotensive subjects receiving diets of 200 or 10 mmol sodium. In the latter studies, blood pressure was measured by a cuff method, which is unlikely to detect the small falls observed in our previous studies (14) where continuous intra-arterial recordings were made. However, infusions of α-hANP were associated with increases in both heart rate and plasma norepinephrine (Fig. 8) when compared with control-day observations. Similar and more marked increases in both heart rate and norepinephrine were observed when α-hANP infusions were given to subjects equilibrated on a low-salt diet. These changes persisted well beyond the disappearance of IR-ANP from plasma (Fig. 8). Although we cannot exclude a direct effect of α-hANP on sympathetic nervous activity, our results from bolus and infusion studies are more consistent with baroreceptor-mediated reflex augmentation of sympathetic activity in response to a minor fall in arterial pressure induced by α-hANP.

In vitro and in vivo experiments indicate that both renin (2) and aldosterone (1) secretion are inhibited by atrial peptides. We found that both PRA

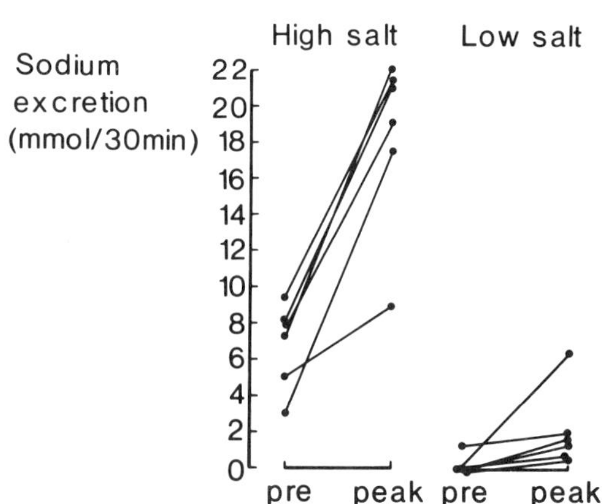

FIG. 7. Urinary sodium excretion immediately before (from 0930 to 1000) and during α-hANP infusions (peak, from 1030 to 1100) in 6 normal subjects studied on high-salt (200 mmol/day) and low-salt (10 mmol/day) intake.

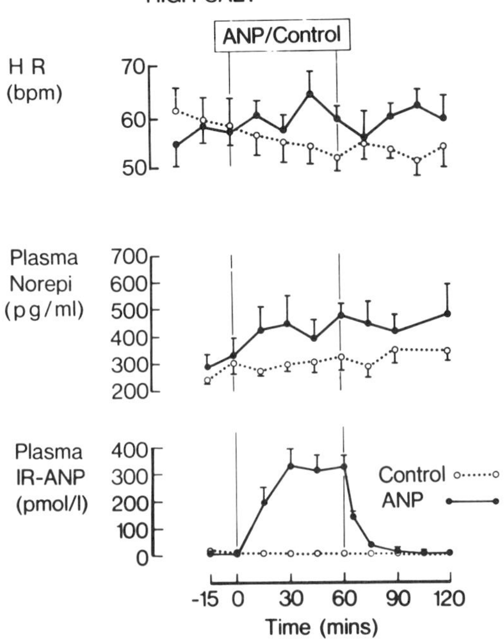

FIG. 8. Response in heart rate (HR, beats per min, *top panel*) and plasma norepinephrine concentrations (*middle panel*) to infusions of α-hANP (*solid line*) and placebo (control, *dotted line*) in 6 normal subjects studied on a daily sodium intake of 200 mmol. Plasma levels of IR-ANP on ANP and control days are also shown. Results are means ± SE. Increase in plasma norepinephrine (compared to placebo day observations) was significant at 0.02 level.

and plasma aldosterone but not cortisol were suppressed during infusions of α-hANP in the normal human. While this inhibition was most apparent when the renin-aldosterone system was activated by prior salt restriction, the percentage decline of both PRA and plasma aldosterone (from preinfusion values) was similar whether the subjects were receiving 200 or 10 mmol sodium (Fig. 9). Plasma angiotensin II concentration was also suppressed by α-hANP in salt-restricted subjects (49 ± 7 pM preinfusion, 28 ± 4 pM postinfusion; $P < 0.008$), whereas levels remained unchanged on the control day (43 ± 9 preinfusion, 42 ± 5 pM postinfusion). This inhibition of the renin-angiotensin-aldosterone axis occurred despite natriuresis and sympathetic activation. Although a significant correlation was noted between maximum decrease in PRA and aldosterone values during infusions of α-hANP, it is not possible to conclude that the fall in aldosterone is necessarily renin dependent. As shown in Figure 9, PRA remained suppressed for 60 min after cessation of α-hANP, during which time plasma aldosterone returned to preinfusion levels. This suggests a more prolonged "after action" of α-hANP on renin than on aldosterone secretion. However, since plasma cortisol also increased in this period in two of six subjects on the low-salt diet, a contribution of ACTH to aldosterone secretion during this postinfusion period cannot be excluded.

In conclusion, both intravenous bolus injections and constant infusions of α-hANP in humans show important actions on electrolyte excretion, hemodynamics, and the renin-angiotensin-aldosterone axis. The natriuretic response appears to depend on both preexisting systemic arterial pressure and sodium status. At plasma concentrations that are observed in some patients

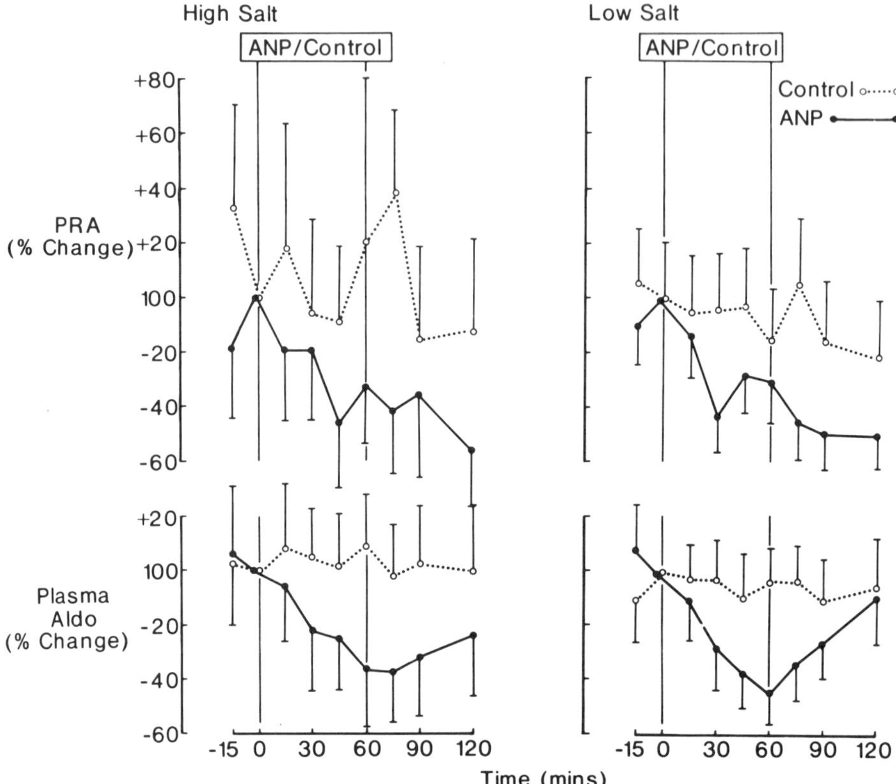

FIG. 9. Percent change in plasma renin activity (PRA) and plasma aldosterone concentration during and after control or α-hANP infusions in 6 normal subjects ingesting 200 mmol sodium/day (*left*) and 10 mmol sodium/day (*right*). Changes (means ± SE) are based on preinfusion levels (100%). On the low-salt diet, the falls in PRA ($P < 0.003$) and aldosterone ($P < 0.007$) at 60 min were highly significant when compared to control day observations.

with cardiovascular disorders, α-hANP increases heart rate and plasma norepinephrine and reduces all elements of the renin-angiotensin-aldosterone system (3). These findings are further support for the view that α-hANP has an important hormonal role in extracellular fluid volume homeostasis in humans.

This research was funded by the National Heart Foundation of New Zealand and the Medical Research Council of New Zealand.

REFERENCES

1. ATARASHI, K., P. J. MULROW, AND R. FRANCO-SAENZ. Effect of atrial peptides on aldosterone production. *J. Clin. Invest.* 76: 1807–1811, 1985.
2. BURNETT, J. C., JR., J. P. GRANGER, AND T. J. OPGENORTH. Effects of synthetic atrial natriuretic factor on renal function and renin release. *Am. J. Physiol.* 247 (*Renal Fluid Electrolyte Physiol.* 16): F863–F866, 1984.

2a. CUNEO, R. C., E. A. ESPINER, M. G. NICHOLLS, T. G. YANDLE, S. L. JOYCE, AND N. L. GILCHRIST. Renal, hemodynamic and hormonal responses to atrial natriuretic peptide infusions in normal man, and effect of sodium intake. *J. Clin. Endocrinol. Metab.* 63: 946–952, 1986.

3. ESPINER, E. A., M. G. NICHOLLS, T. G. YANDLE, I. G. CROZIER, R. C. CUNEO, D. MC-CORMICK, AND H. IKRAM. Studies on the secretion, metabolism and action of atrial natriuretic peptide in man. *J. Hypertens.* 4, Suppl. 2: S85–S91, 1986.

4. FREEMAN, R. H., J. O. DAVIS, AND R. C. VARI. Renal response to atrial natriuretic factor in conscious dogs in caval constriction. *Am. J. Physiol.* 248 (*Regulatory Integrative Comp. Physiol.* 17): R495–R500, 1985.

5. KANGAWA, K., A. FUKUDA, AND H. MATSUO. Structural identification of β- and γ-human atrial natriuretic polypeptides. *Nature Lond.* 313: 397–400, 1985.

6. KIHARA, M., K. NAKAYAMA, K. NAKAO, A. SUGAWARA, N. MORII, M. SAKAMOTO, M. SUDA, M. SHIMOKURA, Y. KISO, H. IMURA, AND Y. YAMORI. Accelerated natriuresis induced by synthetic atrial natriuretic polypeptide in spontaneously hypertensive rats. *Clin. Exp. Hypertens. Part A Theory Pract.* 7: 539–551, 1985.

7. KONDO, K., O. KIDA, K. KANGAWA, H. MATSUO, AND K. TANAKA. Enhanced natriuretic and hypotensive responsiveness to α-human atrial natriuretic polypeptide (α-hANP) in SHR. *Clin. Exp. Hypertens. Part A Theory Pract.* 7: 1097–1107, 1985.

8. LANG, R. E., H. THÖLKEN, D. GANTEN, F. C. LUFT, H. RUSKOAHO, AND T. UNGER. Atrial natriuretic factor—a circulating hormone stimulated by volume loading. *Nature Lond.* 314: 264–266, 1985.

9. MAACK, T., D. N. MARION, M. J. F. CAMARGO, H. D. KLEINERT, J. H. LARAGH, E. D. VAUGHAN, JR., AND S. A. ATLAS. Effects of auriculin (atrial natriuretic factor) on blood pressure, renal function, and the renin-aldosterone system in dogs. *Am. J. Med.* 77: 1069–1075, 1984.

10. MILLAR-CRAIG, M. W., D. HAWES, AND J. WHITTINGTON. New system for recording ambulatory blood pressure in man. *Med. Biol. Eng. Comput.* 16: 727–731, 1978.

11. PANG, S. C., M. C. HOANG, J. TREMBLAY, M. CANTIN, R. GARCIA, J. GENEST, AND P. HAMET. Effect of natural and synthetic atrial natriuretic factor on arterial blood pressure, natriuresis and cyclic GMP excretion in spontaneously hypertensive rats. *Clin. Sci. Mol. Med.* 69: 721–726, 1985.

12. PEGRAM, B. L., M. B. KARDON, N. C. TRIPPODO, F. E. COLE, AND A. A. MACPHEE. Atrial extract: hemodynamics in Wistar-Kyoto and spontaneously hypertensive rats. *Am. J. Physiol.* 249 (*Heart Circ. Physiol.* 18): H265–H271, 1985.

13. RICHARDS, A. M., M. G. NICHOLLS, E. A. ESPINER, H. IKRAM, T. G. YANDLE, S. L. JOYCE, AND M. M. CULLENS. Effects of α-human atrial natriuretic peptide in essential hypertension. *Hypertension Dallas* 7: 812–817, 1985.

14. RICHARDS, A. M., M. G. NICHOLLS, H. IKRAM, M. W. I. WEBSTER, T. G. YANDLE, AND E. A. ESPINER. Renal, haemodynamic, and hormonal effects of human alpha atrial natriuretic peptide in healthy volunteers. *Lancet* 1: 545–549, 1985.

15. SCHWARTZ, D., D. M. GELLER, P. T. MANNING, N. R. SIEGEL, K. F. FOK, C. E. SMITH, AND P. NEEDLEMAN. Ser-Leu-Arg-Arg-atriopeptin III: the major circulating form of atrial peptide. *Science Wash. DC* 229: 397–400, 1985.

16. SEYMOUR, A. A. Renal and systemic effects of atrial natriuretic factor. *Clin. Exp. Hypertens. Part A Theory Pract.* 7: 887–906, 1985.

17. SEYMOUR, A. A., E. A. MARSH, E. K. MAZACK, I. I. STABILITO, AND E. H. BLAINE. Synthetic atrial natriuretic factor in conscious normotensive and hypertensive rats. *Hypertension Dallas* 7, Suppl. I: I35–I42, 1985.

18. YANDLE, T. G., E. A. ESPINER, M. G. NICHOLLS, AND H. DUFF. Radioimmunoassay and characterization of atrial natriuretic peptide in human plasma. *J. Clin. Endocrinol. Metab.* 63: 72–79, 1986.

19. YANDLE, T. G., A. M. RICHARDS, M. G. NICHOLLS, R. C. CUNEO, E. A. ESPINER, AND J. H. LIVESEY. Metabolic clearance rate and plasma half life of alpha human atrial natriuretic peptide in man. *Life Sci.* 38: 1827–1833, 1986.

12

Natriuretic and Sodium-Transport Inhibitory Factors Associated With Volume Control and Hypertension

H. E. DE WARDENER

Research Laboratories, Charing Cross and Westminster
Medical School, London, United Kingdom

ACUTE VOLUME EXPANSION or an increased intake of sodium endows the plasma with an increased capacity to cause a natriuresis, to inhibit sodium transport, and to increase vascular reactivity (23). These changes, which stem from a common stimulus, are due to a change of the concentration in the plasma of at least two substances. One of the substances, a short-acting natriuretic hormone, the atrial natriuretic peptide, does not inhibit sodium transport and diminishes vascular reactivity. Therefore the capacity of the plasma to inhibit sodium transport and to increase vascular reactivity is due to one or more different substances. There are theoretical reasons for suggesting that the plasma's capacity to inhibit sodium transport and to increase vascular reactivity could be due to the same substance (3).

In addition, volume expansion increases the plasma concentration of a long-acting natriuretic substance that has a slow onset (13, 18). When injected into another dehydrated anesthetized rat, 1 ml of plasma from a rat with acute blood volume expansion induces a natriuresis that begins at the end of 1 h and is still increasing at 2 h (Fig. 1; 13). The substance responsible for this slow-onset persisting natriuresis is not known. It is often referred to as the natriuretic hormone. It would perhaps be preferable to call it the long-acting natriuretic hormone. There is some evidence that the long-acting natriuretic hormone has a molecular mass >30,000 (18). Its source is unknown. It has often been assumed that the natriuretic effect of the long-acting natriuretic hormone is caused by the same substance as that which inhibits sodium transport; some authorities have even stated that the natriuretic activity of their extract has been assayed on the frog skin or toad bladder. However, in

127

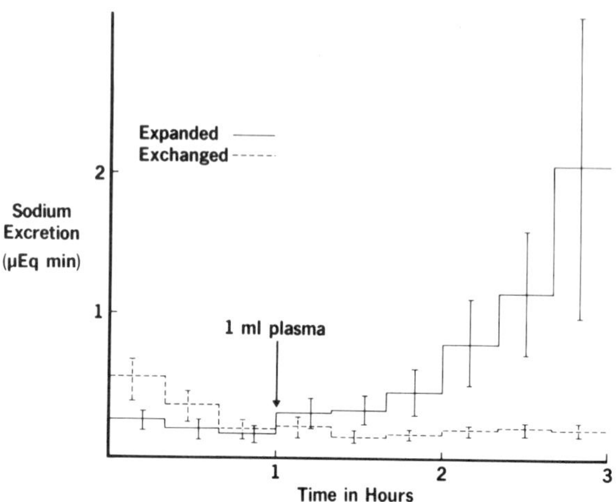

FIG. 1. Mean effect on urinary sodium excretion of a control anesthetized dehydrated 300-g rat of 1 ml plasma from volume-expanded rats and from non-volume-expanded (exchanged) rats. Plasma from urine-reinfused donors; 20 assay rats. [From Knock (13), reprinted by permission from *Clinical Science,* © 1980, The Biochemical Society, London.]

view of the observation that a powerful sodium-transport inhibitor such as ouabain does not cause a natriuresis, except in toxic doses, and that many workers who have attempted to purify the active (natriuretic) substance have only assayed the sodium-transport–inhibiting activity of the material, it is advisable not to assume that the long-acting component of the natriuresis of volume expansion is due to a change in the concentration of the same hormonal substance as that responsible for the sodium-transport–inhibiting activity.

An increased intake of sodium, an acquired persistent difficulty in excreting sodium (e.g., diminution of renal mass), or a brisk change in blood volume causes a change in vascular reactivity due to the presence of a circulating substance. There is no evidence to indicate the site of production of the substance except Jandhyala and Hom's experiment (12), which demonstrates that it does not come from the kidneys (Fig. 2).

PLASMA'S CAPACITY TO INHIBIT NA$^+$-K$^+$-ATPASE ACTIVITY

The increase in the plasma's capacity to inhibit sodium transport, which accompanies volume expansion, was first demonstrated in 1970 (23). More recently it has been considered to be due to a Na^+- and K^+-activated ATPase (Na^+-K^+-ATPase) inhibitor. Recent contributions to this subject have been obtained with a cytochemical bioassay, which detects an Na^+-K^+-ATPase inhibitor. Cytochemical bioassays are in use for several known hormones such as TSH, parathyroid hormone, and gastrin (5). Such assays are based on the principle that when a hormone binds onto its receptor it produces a transient, rapidly reversible effect on an enzyme, which can be revealed by a colored end product at the site of enzymatic activity. Usually a cytochemical bioassay is developed after a protracted search for a suitable enzymatic effect with a pure preparation of the hormone. The specificity of the assay is determined in a variety of ways, including a demonstration that it is competent to distinguish between plasmas with raised and low circulating levels and a demonstration

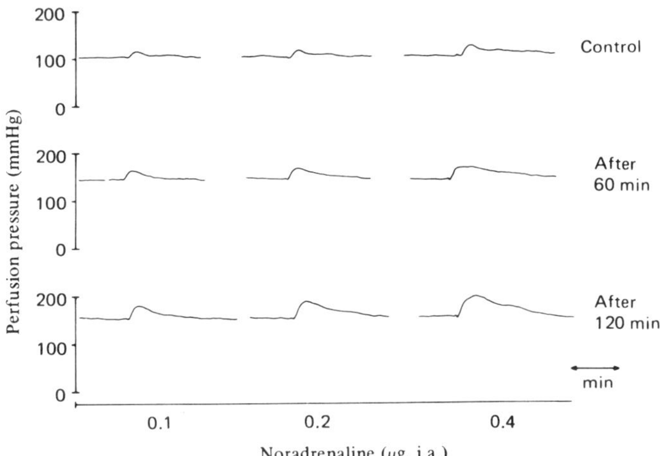

FIG. 2. Polygraph tracings of perfusion-pressure responses to bolus intra-arterial administration (i.a.) of various doses of norepinephrine (noradrenaline) into femoral artery of a denervated
perfused dog hindlimb, before (control) and 60 and 120 min after volume expansion with
equilibrated blood. [From Jandhyala and Hom (12), reprinted by permission from *Clinical Science*,
© 1983, The Biochemical Society, London.]

that the assay is blocked by an antibody to the hormone. In the attempt to
obtain a cytochemical assay for an endogenous Na^+-K^+-ATPase inhibitor the
search was reversed: a predetermined enzymatic effect, inhibition of Na^+-K^+-
ATPase activity, was the starting point that was used to look for an Na^+-K^+-
ATPase inhibitor of unknown structure, the concentration of which, in the
plasma, was controlled by the state of the fluid volume.

The cytochemical technique of Chayen et al. (6) was used to measure
Na^+-K^+-ATPase activity in sections of fresh guinea pig kidney. With this
technique, exposure of a segment of kidney to 4×10^{-4} M ouabain for 2, 4, 6,
and 8 min reveals that ouabain induces a reversible inhibition of Na^+-K^+-
ATPase activity, which is maximal at ~4 min (Fig. 3). In cytochemical assays
of known hormones the time at which a reversible enzymatic effect is maximal
is one of the features that confers specificity. Dilutions of normal plasma also
induce a reversible inhibition of Na^+-K^+-ATPase activity with a maximal
effect at ~4–6 min (Fig. 3). With this technique it was found that plasma from
salt-loaded humans inhibited Na^+-K^+-ATPase activity ~25 times more than
when the plasma was obtained from the same individuals on a low-sodium
diet (Fig. 4; 25).

PLASMA'S ABILITY TO STIMULATE GLUCOSE-6-PHOSPHATE
DEHYDROGENASE ACTIVITY

The cytochemical technique with which Na^+-K^+-ATPase–inhibiting activity is measured is semiquantitative. It is possible to obtain some information
from the time course, but the small amount of Na^+-K^+-ATPase activity

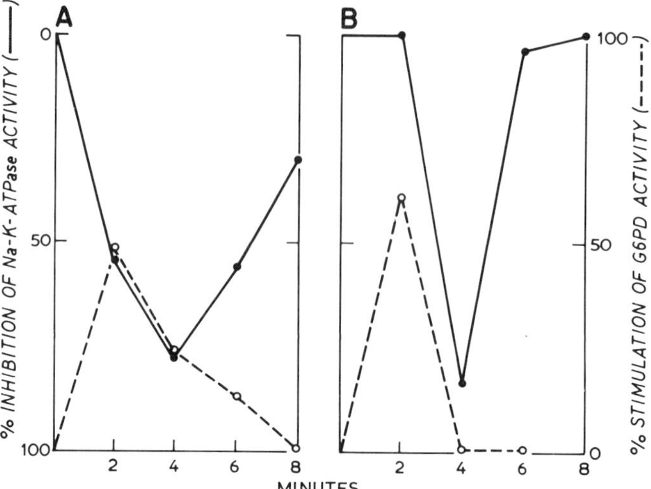

FIG. 3. Percentage changes in glucose-6-phosphate dehydrogenase (G6PD) and Na$^+$-K$^+$-ATPase activity in proximal tubules of segments of fresh guinea pig kidney exposed to 1/1,000 plasma (A) or 4 × 10^{-4} M ouabain (B) for 2 to 8 min, measured with cytochemical techniques.

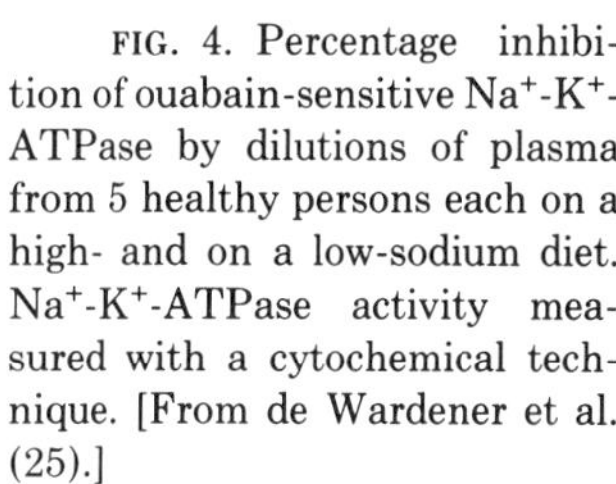

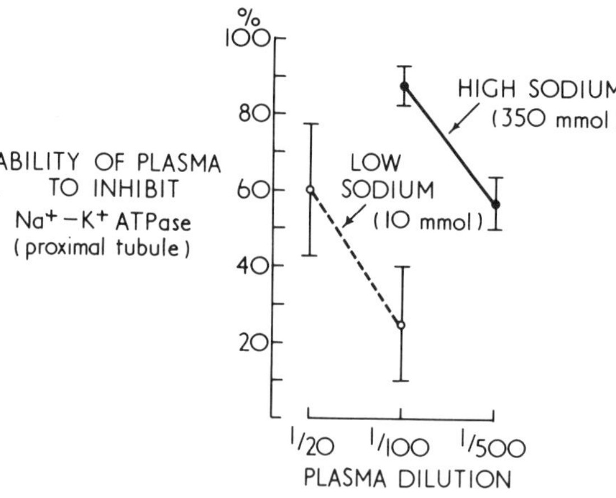

FIG. 4. Percentage inhibition of ouabain-sensitive Na$^+$-K$^+$-ATPase by dilutions of plasma from 5 healthy persons each on a high- and on a low-sodium diet. Na$^+$-K$^+$-ATPase activity measured with a cytochemical technique. [From de Wardener et al. (25).]

remaining in the kidney section has, until recently, made it difficult to obtain a dose-response curve of sufficient steepness, with a standard, to validate a reproducible and precise quantitative assay. Inhibition of Na$^+$-K$^+$-ATPase, however, in fresh tissue is associated with stimulation of glucose-6-phosphate dehydrogenase (G6PD) activity (7). The metabolic connection between the two enzymes is unclear; a change in the state of glutathione or the involvement of certain arachidonic acid metabolites has been suggested. The cytochemical technique used to measure G6PD activity quantitatively is well established. With this technique, exposure of guinea pig kidney for 2–8 min to 4 × 10^{-4} M ouabain induces a reversible rise in G6PD activity, which is maximal at 2 min (Fig. 3). Normal plasma also induces a reversible stimulation of G6PD, which is maximal at 2 min (Fig. 3). The time course of the fall in Na$^+$-K$^+$-ATPase activity and rise in G6PD activity in kidney segments exposed to plasma is usually measured in separate segments of guinea pig kidney in separate experiments, but the effect of the plasma on the two enzymes in the same segment of kidney has also been studied. After exposure to the plasma for 2, 4, 6, and 8 min, alternate sections from a segment were either prepared to demonstrate Na^+-K^+-ATPase activity or to demonstrate G6PD activity. It was then possible to observe that G6PD activity in the segments is maximal after 2 min of exposure to plasma and falls to normal by 6 min, whereas Na^+-K^+-ATPase activity in the segment begins to fall at 2 min, is lowest at 4–6 min, and then returns toward control values.

The dose-response curve of the effect of dilutions of plasma on G6PD activity after 2 min of exposure is linear and sufficiently steep to give reproducible results. This has enabled development and validation of a precise quantitative assay that measures the capacity of body fluids, or extracts, to stimulate G6PD at 2 min as an index of their ability to inhibit Na^+-K^+-ATPase (10). A high-potency plasma is used as standard. In established cytochemical bioassays for known hormones the quantitative effect induced by a pure hormone is only evident over a specific range of low concentrations of the hormone. With increasing dilutions of the high-potency plasma, the stimulation of G6PD activity at 2 min becomes evident, reaches a peak of activity, and then returns to base line in a log-linear relationship (Fig. 5). It is the linearity and reproducibility of this return of G6PD-stimulating activity to zero that endows the assay with precision. The amount of G6PD stimulation that produces maximum G6PD stimulation at 2 min is defined as one unit of G6PD-stimulating activity. The use of a standard to quantify the G6PD-stimulating activity of an unknown assumes that the activity of the unknown is due to the same material as that which causes the activity in the standard;

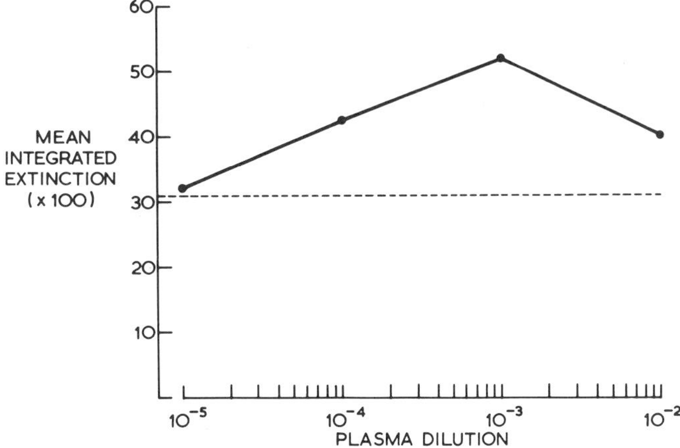

FIG. 5. Changes in G6PD activity as shown by amount of formazan deposit measured by microdensitometry expressed as mean integrated extinction in proximal tubules in segments of guinea pig kidney exposed for 2 min to dilutions of a high-potency plasma. – – – – – , G6PD activity in a segment exposed to culture medium alone.

therefore the assay can only be quantitative if the dose-response curve of the unknown is parallel to that of the standard.

The intra-assay variation of this bioassay is within 10% and the interassay variation is within 22%, with a mean index of precision for nine consecutive assays of 0.07 ± 0.004, which is well within the accepted limits for bioassays. Tests of specificity have been performed with many substances known to act on the nephron, including aldosterone, angiotensin II, vasopressin, dopamine, norepinephrine, epinephrine, parathyroid hormone, calcitonin, 1,25-dihydroxyvitamin D, thyrotropin-releasing hormone, luteinizing hormone, and, more recently, linoleic acid, oleic acid, dehydroepiandrosterone-sulfate, lysophosphatidal choline, and sodium vanadate. None stimulates G6PD activity at 2 min.

CYTOCHEMICAL TECHNIQUES

Female guinea pigs of the Duncan-Hartley strain weighing 300–450 g are killed by cervical fracture and both kidneys are removed, cut into segments, and placed in sealed pots in a nonproliferative culture medium under an atmosphere of 95% O_2-5% CO_2 at 37°C for 5 h. The medium is then replaced with fresh medium containing various dilutions of plasma for 2–8 min (depending on which of the two assays is being used). The segments are chilled by immersion in n-hexane ($-70°C$), and 16-μm-thick sections are cut from each segment with a cryostat microtome at $-30°C$. To demonstrate G6PD activity the sections are incubated at 37°C under an atmosphere of nitrogen in a reaction medium containing G6PD (5 mM), the coenzyme NADP (3 mM), neotetrazolium chloride (5 mM), potassium cyanide (10 mM), phenazine methosulfate (0.67 mM), and polyvinyl alcohol (G18 12% wt/vol) dissolved in a 0.05 mM glycylglycine sodium hydroxide buffer (pH 8.2). The reaction is stopped by immersing the sections in distilled water. The activity of the G6PD is shown by the deposition of an intensely colored, highly localized formazan. A plasma of high potency is used as a standard.

To demonstrate Na^+-K^+-ATPase activity the sections from tissue segments are preincubated at 37°C in a medium containing 40% (wt/vol) polypeptide (Polypep 5115 Sigma) and 0.1 M potassium acetate dissolved in 0.2 M Tris at pH 7.4 for 2 min to remove free phosphate. The preincubation buffer is then replaced for 15 min by reaction medium containing 40% (wt/vol) polypeptide, potassium chloride (37.5 mM), sodium chloride (410 mM), magnesium chloride (20 mM), ATP (10 mM), sodium acetate (2 mM), together with lead ammonium citrate and acetate complex (32 g/liter) (previously dissolved by shaking in the smallest amounts of dilute ammonia) and dissolved in 0.2 M Tris buffer at pH 7.4. The sections are rinsed several times in 0.2 M Tris buffer at pH 7.4 and immersed in water saturated with H_2S for 2 min. This procedure demonstrates the total ATPase activity as a brown precipitate. The Na^+-K^+-ATPase (i.e., ouabain-sensitive ATPase) is determined by including ouabain (2×10^{-4} M) in the reaction medium in serial sections, then subtracting the ouabain-insensitive ATPase activity from the total ATPase activity. The colored reaction products of the enzymes are measured with a Vickers M8S scanning and integrating microdensitometer at a wavelength of 585 nm and a magnification of 400 in 20 proximal tubules from duplicate sections from each segment. Statistical assessment of assay validity and potency ratios have been made with reference to the *European Pharmacopoeia* (9).

The ability of plasma to stimulate G6PD is severely depressed by freezing and thawing on more than one occasion, while it is increased >100% by heating at 37°C for 15 min. It is diminished >90% by heating at 37°C for 45 min. These effects are not influenced by aprotinin. The plasma's activity survives heating at 100°C for 10 min, and the activity of the supernate obtained from this procedure survives heating at 105°C in 6 N HCl for 18 h and passes through an Amicon UM05 ultrafiltration membrane, suggesting a molecular weight <500. The activity of the plasma supernate is diminished >80% by incubation with digoxin antibody. Note that the only connections that have been found with the substance in the plasma that inhibits Na^+-K^+-ATPase and stimulates G6PD are the glycosides ouabain and digoxin.

The effect of salt intake on the plasma's ability to stimulate G6PD was studied in normal subjects and normal rats on low- and high-sodium intakes. The plasma's ability to stimulate G6PD when obtained from humans and rats on high-sodium diets was 39.6 ± 10.6 and 33.1 ± 5.8 G6PD-stimulating units per milliliter, respectively, and on the low-salt diet it was 1.83 ± 0.5 and 5.0 G6PD-stimulating units per milliliter (Fig. 6).

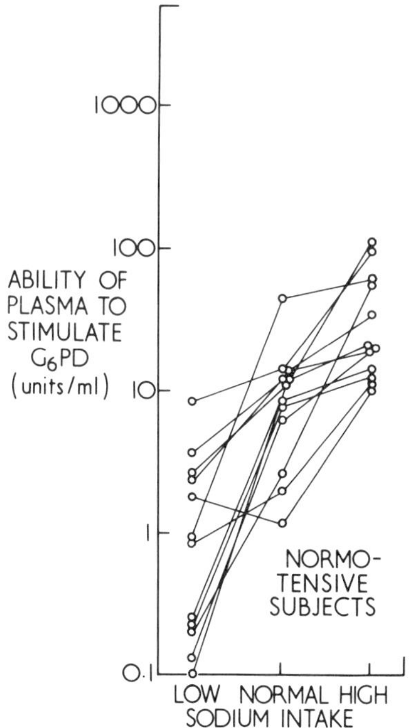

FIG. 6. Ability of plasma from 12 normal subjects on a low-, normal-, and high-sodium intake to stimulate G6PD activity. G6PD activity is measured with a cytochemical bioassay. [Adapted from Fenton et al. (10).]

HYPOTHALAMUS

To find the source of the plasma Na^+-K^+-ATPase inhibitor, acetone extracts were prepared from the pituitary gland, cerebral cortex, muscle, heart, adrenal gland, liver, spleen, pancreas, kidney, stomach, duodenum, jejunum, ileum, and hypothalamus. The extracts were assayed for their cytochemical bioassayable ability to inhibit Na^+-K^+-ATPase activity directly, and indirectly by their capacity to stimulate G6PD activity. Acetone extracts of hypothalamus contained large quantities of Na^+-K^+-ATPase–inhibiting and G6PD-stimulating activity. The G6PD-stimulating activity from one hypothalamus is ~10,000–100,000 times greater than that of 1 ml of plasma. It was also found that the content of G6PD-stimulating activity in the hypothalamus of the normal rat is influenced by the animal's salt intake. The content of G6PD-stimulating activity of a hypothalamic extract from rats that had been fed a high-sodium diet for 4 wk was $419.6 \pm 110 \times 10^4$ G6PD-stimulating units per hypothalamus and $2.56 \pm 0.59 \times 10^4$ G6PD-stimulating units per hypothalamus when obtained from rats on a low-sodium diet for 4 wk. The G6PD-stimulating activity obtained from the hypothalamus has the same properties as those of the plasma. It survives boiling for 10 min and 6 N HCl for 18 h at 105°C under nitrogen, it passes through an Amicon UM05 ultrafiltration membrane, and it is inhibited >80% by digoxin antibody. It is also destroyed by exposure to pH 12 for 3 h at room temperature. These many similarities, including the fact that both the plasma and hypothalamic extract inhibit Na^+-K^+-ATPase at 4–6 min and stimulate G6PD at 2 min in the cytochemical bioassays and that the dose-response curves of the plasma and hypothalamic extract are parallel, suggest that the Na^+-K^+-ATPase–inhibiting and G6PD-stimulating substance in the plasma and hypothalamus may be the same.

An attempt was made to extract and purify the active material from the rat hypothalamus. The animals were killed by decapitation and the hypothalami removed. The hypothalami were homogenized in 1 ml of acetone and placed on a rotary mixer for 3 h at 37°C. The acetone extract was then centrifuged and the acetone-soluble fraction dried with nitrogen. The residue was then dissolved in acid water (pH 3) and treated with chloroform, as the activity was insoluble in chloroform. The acid water was then placed onto silica gel thin-layer electrophoresis when the activity appeared in a relatively circumscribed fraction well beyond a lysine marker. The activity was extracted from the silica gel with methanol and placed on reverse-phase high-performance liquid chromatography (HPLC) when the activity appeared in a discrete fraction that had no UV absorption. Plasma supernate, after boiling for 10 min, was extracted in the same manner; the Na^+-K^+-ATPase–inhibiting and G6PD-stimulating activity appeared in the same fractions as the hypothalamic activity, adding further support to the proposition that the Na^+-K^+-ATPase inhibitor in the plasma and hypothalamus may be the same (1).

HYPERTENSION

The plasma concentration of atrial natriuretic peptide is raised in essential hypertension (20) and the Dahl salt-sensitive rat (22), while in the spontaneously hypertensive rat (SHR) there is a reduction in the atrial content of natriuretic peptide (21). The ability of plasma to increase vascular reactivity is raised in essential hypertension (24) and the SHR (26). The plasma from patients suffering from essential hypertension (16) and plasma from the SHR (17) and the Milan hypertensive rat (2) have an increased Na^+-K^+-ATPase–inhibiting and G6PD-stimulating activity. These three changes are a normal feature of acute volume expansion or a raised dietary intake of sodium.

ESSENTIAL HYPERTENSION

The ouabain-sensitive sodium-efflux rate constant of leukocytes in essential hypertension is reduced and inversely correlated with the arterial pressure (11) but is directly correlated with plasma renin activity. That this effect is due to a circulating substance is demonstrated by incubating leukocytes from normotensive subjects in the plasma of hypertensive patients when the ouabain-sensitive sodium-efflux rate constant of the normal leukocytes falls to the same levels as those of the patients' own leukocytes (Fig. 7; 11, 19). Theoretically a rise in the plasma concentration of an Na^+-K^+-ATPase inhibitor should raise the concentration of intracellular sodium and thus the intracellular calcium concentration (3). It is possible therefore that the rise in platelet calcium that has been described in patients with essential hypertension and in the SHR, which is directly correlated with the arterial pressure (4, 8), is due to the circulating sodium-transport inhibitor. As with leukocytes, a rise in platelet calcium can be induced in platelets of normotensive subjects by incubation in the plasma of hypertensive patients (14).

The ability of plasma from patients with essential hypertension to stimulate G6PD activity at 2 min was 195 ± 52 G6PD-stimulating units per milliliter, which was significantly higher than that of normotensive subjects in whom it was 22.5 ± 5.8 G6PD-stimulating units per milliliter (Fig. 8; 16). When the two groups were combined there was a significant correlation between the arterial pressure and the ability of the plasma to stimulate G6PD activity. In patients with a low plasma renin (0.5 $\mu g \cdot ml^{-1} \cdot h^{-1}$) it was 400 ±

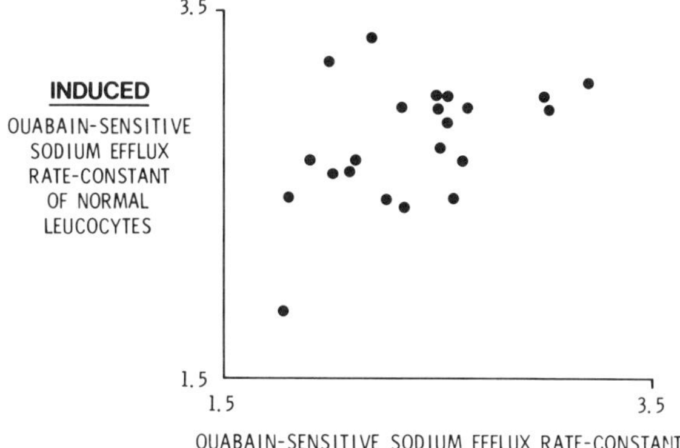

FIG. 7. Induced ouabain-sensitive sodium-efflux rate constant of leukocytes from normotensive individuals after incubation in plasma of hypertensive patients plotted against the ouabain-sensitive sodium-efflux rate constant of the hypertensive patient's own leukocytes. [Adapted from Hilton (11).]

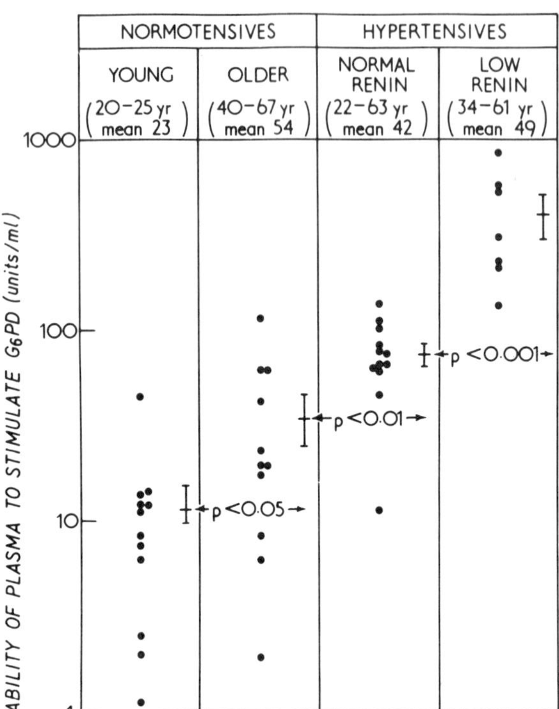

FIG. 8. Ability of plasma to stimulate G6PD in a young and an older group of normotensive subjects and in 2 groups of hypertensive patients. Both normotensives and hypertensives on a normal-sodium diet. One hypertensive group had normal plasma renin activity; the other had low plasma renin activity. [From MacGregor et al. (16), reprinted by permission from *Clinical Science*, © 1981, The Biochemical Society, London.]

97 G6PD-stimulating units per milliliter, which was significantly higher than in hypertensive patients with a normal plasma renin in whom it was 74.9 ± 9.2 G6PD-stimulating units per milliliter, though this was significantly greater than the normotensive subjects. In hypertensive patients the ability of plasma to stimulate G6PD activity at 2 min was inversely correlated with plasma renin activity, but not in the normotensive subjects. In five hypertensive patients the ability of the plasma to stimulate G6PD activity when they were on a low-sodium intake (<10 mmol/day) was 380 ± 96 G6PD-stimulating units per milliliter in contrast to 980 ± 303 G6PD-stimulating units per milliliter when they were on a high-sodium intake (>300 mmol/day).

SPONTANEOUSLY HYPERTENSIVE RAT

In the adult SHR and in the Wistar-Kyoto (WKY) rat normotensive control, the plasma's ability to stimulate G6PD at 2 min was 772.3 ± 48.1 G6PD-stimulating units per milliliter and 12.5 ± 2.6 G6PD-stimulating units per milliliter, respectively (17). The content of G6PD-stimulating activity in an acetone extract of the hypothalamus of the SHR was $2.2 \pm 1.7 \times 10^8$ units, and in the hypothalamus of the WKY it was $4.5 \pm 1.8 \times 10^4$ units. The SHR hypothalamus therefore appears to contain ~1,000 times more G6PD-stimulating activity than that of a normal rat. For this reason the SHR hypothalamus is now used as source material for extraction and purification procedures.

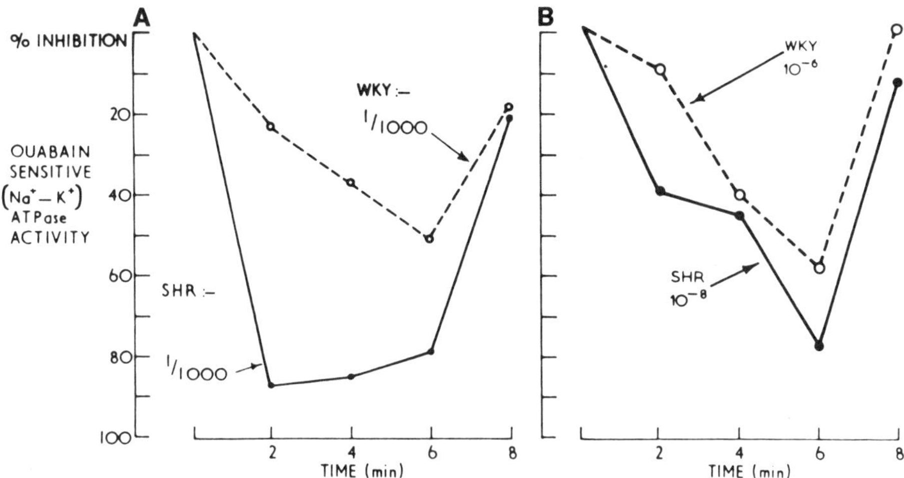

FIG. 9. Percentage inhibition of Na⁺-K⁺-ATPase activity of fresh guinea pig kidney proximal tubules exposed for 2, 4, 6, and 8 min to plasma dilutions (*A*) and hypothalamic extracts (*B*) from spontaneously hypertensive (SHR) and normotensive Wistar-Kyoto (WKY) rats, with a cyto-chemical bioassay used to measure Na⁺-K⁺-ATPase activity. [From Millett et al. (17).]

With the semiquantitative assay, which measures the Na⁺-K⁺-ATPase activity directly, plasma and acetone extracts of hypothalamus from the SHR had a greater capacity to inhibit Na⁺-K⁺-ATPase at 4–6 min than the plasma and hypothalamus of the WKY rat (Fig. 9). The observation that in the SHR the ability of the plasma and the hypothalamus to inhibit Na⁺-K⁺-ATPase activity and to stimulate G6PD activity are both raised supports the proposition that the hypothalamus may be the source of the substance in the plasma.

MILAN HYPERTENSIVE RAT

Recently Alaghband-Zadeh et al. (2) measured the cytochemically assay-able Na⁺-K⁺-ATPase–inhibiting and G6PD-stimulating activity of the plasma of the 3- and 9-wk-old Milan hypertensive rat and of their normotensive control. At 3 wk the blood pressure of the hypertensive-strain rat is normal; at 9 wk the rat is hypertensive. The ability of plasma from the normotensive 3-wk hypertensive-strain rat and its normotensive control was 99.9 ± 27.4 and 7.8 ± 1.8 G6PD-stimulating units per milliliter, respectively; in the 9-wk rat it was 586.0 ± 88 and 23.4 ± 8.3 G6PD-stimulating units per milliliter, respectively. With the semiquantitative Na⁺-K⁺-ATPase assay the plasma from the 9-wk hypertensive-strain rat had a greater capacity to inhibit Na⁺-K⁺-ATPase than the plasma of the 9-wk normotensive rat. The plasma's capacity to stimulate G6PD activity at 3 wk of age in the hypertensive strain of rat, before the main rise in arterial pressure had occurred, suggests that the rise in Na⁺-K⁺-ATPase–inhibiting and G6PD-stimulating ability of the plasma at 9 wk, when the rat is hypertensive, is not a secondary phenomenon related to the rise in arterial pressure or to the effect of the hypertension on renal

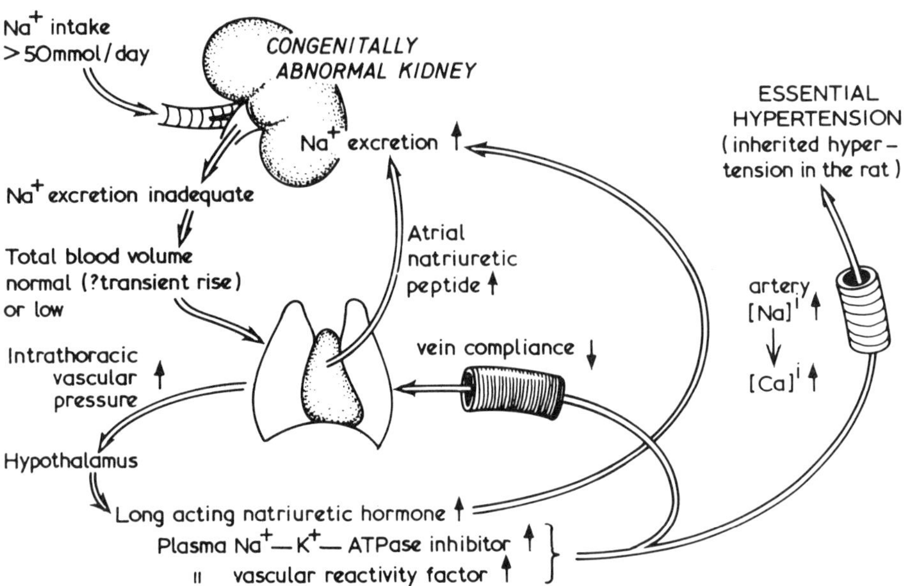

FIG. 10. Schema of hypothesis for rise in arterial pressure in inherited hypertension.

function. It also suggests that the substance responsible for the inhibition of
Na⁺-K⁺-ATPase activity and stimulation of G6PD activity may be involved
in the rise in arterial pressure.

Recently we have found that the G6PD-stimulating activity of the plasma
from hypertensive patients, the SHR, and the Milan hypertensive rat is
suppressed >80% by digoxin antibody. This finding, together with the observation that the plasma in these conditions also inhibits Na⁺-K⁺-ATPase at 4–
6 min, stimulates G6PD at 2 min, and has a dose-response curve parallel to
that of the normal human and the rat, suggests that the inhibitory substance
in these three forms of hereditary hypertension and in the normal human and
the rat is the same.

HYPOTHESIS

These various changes in these three forms of hereditary hypertension
can also be observed in normal subjects on a high-sodium intake. Their
presence in hereditary forms of hypertension, and therefore in patients and
rats on a normal-sodium intake, suggests that in these hereditary forms of
hypertension there is a persistent tendency to retain sodium. This suggestion
dovetails with recent evidence that in essential hypertension, the SHR, and
the Milan hypertensive rat, proximal tubule sodium reabsorption is increased.
This abnormality may be due to an increase in Na⁺-H⁺ countertransport and
is probably a local manifestation of a generalized genetic abnormality of plasma
membranes that, in the erythrocytes of patients with essential hypertension,

is evident as the well-documented increase in Na^+-Na^+ (Na^+-Li^+) counter-transport.

The presence of a renal sodium-retaining lesion and evidence in the plasma that is compatible with a persistent tendency to retain sodium in these three forms of hereditary hypertension are curious findings, inasmuch as it is well established that the total blood volume in inherited forms of hypertension is usually normal or low, and inversely correlated with the blood pressure. Nevertheless, though the blood volume in hereditary forms of hypertension is low, it is increasingly evident that intrathoracic vascular pressures are raised. It is proposed that it is this rise that not only causes the rise in plasma atrial natriuretic peptide but is also responsible for the plasma's increased ability to inhibit Na^+-K^+-ATPase activity and to increase vascular reactivity. Initially the rise in these intrathoracic vascular pressures is probably caused by a transient retention of sodium and increase in extracellular fluid volume, a phenomenon that has frequently been observed as the blood pressure is rising in hypertensive strains of young rats. Later, when the hypertension is established and the blood volume is normal or low, it is probable that the rise in central venous pressure is due, as London et al. (15) propose, to the well-documented decrease in the compliance of the peripheral venous system—a diminution that does not appear to be due to cardiac hypertrophy or cardiac failure and that can be demonstrated in the forearm veins. This is an abnormality that has been noted in all forms of hypertension. Presumably it is due to the same disturbance of the smooth muscle of the veins as that which affects the smooth muscle of the arterioles and causes the rise in arterial pressure. The nature of this abnormality is not known, but there are good theoretical reasons for suggesting that it may be related to the plasma's increased ability to inhibit Na^+-K^+-ATPase and to increase vascular reactivity (3).

In summary (Fig. 10) it is proposed that in inherited forms of hypertension a genetic abnormality of the Na^+-H^+ exchange in the proximal tubule causes an increased sodium reabsorption, the effect of which is more pronounced the higher the salt intake. Initially this causes a transient increase in total blood volume and central venous pressure, which increases plasma atrial natriuretic peptide and stimulates the hypothalamus to increase the secretion of long-acting natriuretic hormone and the factors responsible for the plasma's ability to inhibit Na^+-K^+-ATPase and to increase vascular reactivity. Sodium balance is restored but at the cost of a persistently raised level of natriuretic, Na^+-K^+-ATPase–inhibiting, and vascular reactivity factors. The latter influence the vascular smooth muscle of the arteries (which causes the rise in arterial pressure) and the smooth muscle of the veins (which diminishes venous compliance). The diminution in venous compliance raises intrathoracic vascular pressures, which perpetuates the stimulus for the increase in the plasma's concentration of the short- and long-acting natriuretic substances, the Na^+-K^+-ATPase and the vascular reactivity factor, even if the blood volume falls to below normal.

It is also suggested that in most forms of experimental or secondary hypertension the sequence of events leading to the rise in arterial pressure is similar except that the tendency to retain sodium is more obvious. It is acquired in disease or imposed by an experimental surgical procedure (e.g., reduced renal mass, clipping of renal arteries) or by the administration of a salt-retaining hormone such as deoxycorticosterone acetate.

This work was supported by grants from the Medical Research Council, the National Kidney Research Fund, the British Heart Foundation, and the Fondation Clarisse Neiman.

REFERENCES

1. ALAGHBAND-ZADEH, J., S. FENTON, K. HANCOCK, J. MILLETT, AND H. E. DE WARDENER. Evidence that the hypothalamus may be a source of a circulating Na$^+$-K$^+$-ATPase inhibitor. *J. Endocrinol.* 98: 221–226, 1983.
2. ALAGHBAND-ZADEH, J., S. M. HOLLAND, J. A. MILLETT, H. E. DE WARDENER, P. FERRARI, AND G. BIANCHI. Increased circulating Na$^+$-K$^+$-ATPase inhibitor in the young and adult Milan hypertensive strain rat. *Clin. Sci. Lond.* 70, Suppl. 13: 58p, 1986.
3. BLAUSTEIN, M. P. Sodium ions, calcium ions, blood pressure regulation, and hypertension: a reassessment and a hypothesis. *Am. J. Physiol.* 232 (*Cell Physiol.* 1): C165–C173, 1977.
4. BRUSCHI, G., M. E. BRUSCHI, M. CAROPPO, G. ORLANDINI, M. SPAGGIARI, AND A. CAVA-TORTA. Cytoplasmic free [Ca^{2+}] is increased in the platelets of spontaneously hypertensive rats and essential hypertensive patients. *Clin Sci. Lond.* 68: 179–184, 1985.
5. CHAYEN, J., AND L. BITENSKY. *Cytochemical Bioassays: Techniques and Applications.* New York: Dekker, 1983.
6. CHAYEN, J., G. T. FROST, R. A. DODDS, L. BITENSKY, J. PITCHFORK, P. H. BAYLIS, AND R. J. BARNETT. The use of a hidden metal-capture reagent for the measurement of Na$^+$-K$^+$-ATPase activity: a new concept in cytochemistry. *Histochemistry* 71: 533–541, 1981.
7. DIKSTEIN, S. Stimulability, adenosine triphosphatases and their control by cellular redox processes. *Naturwissenschaften* 58: 439–443, 1971.
8. ERNE, P., P. BOLLI, E. BÜRGISSER, AND F. R. BÜHLER. Correlation of platelet calcium with blood pressure. Effect of antihypertensive therapy. *N. Engl. J. Med.* 310: 1084–1088, 1984.
9. Council of Europe. *European Pharmacopoeia. II. Statistical Analysis of Results of Biological Assays and Tests.* Strasbourg, France: Maisonneuve, 1971.
10. FENTON, S., E. CLARKSON, G. MACGREGOR, J. ALAGHBAND-ZADEH, AND H. E. DE WARDE-NER. An assay of the capacity of biological fluids to stimulate renal glucose-6-phosphate dehydrogenase activity in vitro as a marker of their ability to inhibit sodium potassium-dependent adenosine triphosphatase activity. *J. Endocrinol.* 94: 99–110, 1982.
11. HILTON, P. J. Factors influencing leucocyte sodium transport in hypertension. *Klin. Wochenschr.* 63, Suppl. 3: 49–51, 1985.
12. JANDHYALA, B. S., AND G. J. HOM. Effects of acute blood volume expansion on vascular resistance and reactivity in anaesthetised dogs. *Clin. Sci. Lond.* 65: 9–17, 1983.
13. KNOCK, C. A. Further evidence in vivo for a circulating natriuretic substance after expanding the blood volume in rats. *Clin. Sci. Lond.* 59: 423–433, 1980.
14. LINDNER, A., H. PARK, AND M. KENNEY. Circulating plasma factor in essential hypertension raises intracellular free calcium in normal platelets (abstr.). *Kidney Int.* 29: 250, 1986.
15. LONDON, G. M., M. E. SAFAR, A. E. SAFAR, AND A. C. SIMON. Blood pressure in the "low pressure" system and cardiac performance in essential hypertension. *J. Hypertens.* 3: 337–342, 1985.
16. MACGREGOR, G. A., S. FENTON, J. ALAGHBAND-ZADEH, N. D. MARKANDU, J. E. ROULSTON, AND H. E. DE WARDENER. An increase in a circulating inhibitor of Na$^+$,K$^+$-dependent ATPase: a possible link between salt intake and the development of essential hypertension. *Clin. Sci. Lond.* 61, Suppl. 7: 17s–20s, 1981.
17. MILLETT, J. A., S. M. HOLLAND, J. ALAGHBAND-ZADEH, AND H. E. DE WARDENER. Na$^+$-K$^+$-ATPase-inhibiting and glucose-6-phosphate dehydrogenase-stimulating activity of plasma and hypothalamus of the Okamoto spontaneously hypertensive rat. *J. Endocrinol.* 108: 69–73, 1986.
18. PEARCE, J. W., AND A. T. VERESS. Concentration and bioassay of a natriuretic factor in plasma of volume expanded rats. *Can. J. Physiol. Pharmacol.* 53: 742–747, 1975.

19. POSTON, L., R. B. SEWELL, S. P. WILKINSON, P. J. RICHARDSON, R. WILLIAMS, E. M. CLARKSON, G. A. MACGREGOR, AND H. E. DE WARDENER. Evidence for a circulating sodium transport inhibitor in essential hypertension. *Br. Med. J.* 282: 847–849, 1981.

20. SAGNELLA, G. A., N. D. MARKANDU, A. C. SHORE, AND G. A. MACGREGOR. Raised circulating levels of atrial natriuretic peptides in essential hypertension. *Lancet* 1: 179–181, 1986.

21. SONNENBERG, H., S. MILOJEVIC, C. K. CHONG, AND A. T. VERESS. Atrial natriuretic factor: reduced cardiac content in spontaneously hypertensive rats. *Hypertension Dallas* 5: 672–675, 1983.

22. TANAKA, I., AND T. INAGAMI. Increased concentration of plasma immunoreactive ANF in salt sensitive rats with NaCl induced hypertension. *J. Hypertens.* 4: 109–112, 1986.

23. WARDENER, H. E. DE, AND E. M. CLARKSON. Concept of natriuretic hormone. *Physiol. Rev.* 65: 658–759, 1985.

24. WARDENER, H. E. DE, AND G. A. MACGREGOR. The relation of a circulating sodium transport inhibitor (the natriuretic hormone?) to hypertension. *Medicine Baltimore* 62: 310–326, 1983.

25. WARDENER, H. E. DE, G. A. MACGREGOR, E. M. CLARKSON, J. ALAGHBAND-ZADEH, L. BITENSKY, AND J. CHAYEN. Effect of sodium intake on ability of human plasma to inhibit renal Na^+-K^+-adenosine triphosphatase in vitro. *Lancet* 1: 411–413, 1981.

26. WRIGHT, G. L. The vascular sensitizing character of plasma from spontaneously hypertensive rats. *Can. J. Physiol. Pharmacol.* 59: 1111–1116, 1981.

13

Endogenous Sodium-Transport Inhibitors as Physiological Regulators of the Sodium Pump

GARNER T. HAUPERT, JR.

Renal Unit, Massachusetts General Hospital, Harvard Medical School, Boston, Massachusetts

SINCE THE DISCOVERY of endogenous analogues of opium, the endorphins and enkephalins (16, 27), it has been tempting to postulate that parallel situations might obtain for other pharmacologically potent substances from the plant kingdom that exert their effects through specific receptors in animal tissues. Thus the Na^+- and K^+-activated ATPase (Na^+-K^+-ATPase) in animal species might have an endogenous analogue to the cardiac glycosides. Several "endogenous factors" that either inhibit active sodium transport, inhibit Na^+-K^+-ATPase activity in vitro, or prevent ouabain binding to the Na^+-K^+-ATPase have been extracted from amphibian and mammalian sources (for a review, see ref. 12). Such an endogenous sodium-transport inhibitor has been implicated in many important physiological and pathophysiological processes. De Wardener et al. (30) suggested that the natriuresis of intravascular volume expansion was mediated in part by a humoral substance distinct from known regulators of renal hemodynamics and tubular cation transport. Hillyard et al. (15) recognized the ouabainlike effects of such a substance during their attempts to characterize a natriuretic principle extracted from renal tissue of volume-expanded rats. At about the same time Overbeck et al. (21) showed that volume expansion was associated with the elaboration of a heat-stable substance in plasma that inhibited cell membrane sodium transport in vascular muscle, and Haddy and Overbeck (9) postulated that the unknown compound might be responsible for the sequence of physiological events characterizing the development of experimental volume-expanded hypertension in animals. A decrease in sodium-pump activity was documented in uremia (7, 31), and a natriuretic factor was found in the urine of uremic patients with intravascular

143

volume expansion but not in that of nephrotic uremics who demonstrate the physiology of intravascular volume depletion (2). It was hypothesized that this factor might be important in the adaptive response to progressive nephron loss whereby an enhanced fractional excretion of sodium permits maintenance of normal sodium balance in patients with nonnephrotic chronic renal failure (23). It also seems that patients with essential hypertension have an elevated concentration of a circulating pump inhibitor (6, 11, 22), raising the provocative possibility that an abnormality in regulation of Na^+-K^+-ATPase plays a role in a prevalent human disease.

This background of both experimental and clinical observations has stimulated a concerted effort by many laboratories to isolate and identify the endogenous Na^+-K^+-ATPase inhibitor. Though considerable effort has been expended over many years, a purified substance of known structure is not in hand. Considerable controversy still exists even as to the chemical nature of the substance; some maintain it is a peptide; others affirm properties that are manifestly inconsistent with this class of compounds (12). Remember, however, that vertebrates are able to synthesize substances closely analogous in structure and pharmacological properties to the digitalis glycosides. The bufodienolides, present in the skin of certain toads, are, like the digitalis glycosides, steroid-lactone compounds that inhibit Na^+-K^+-ATPase (8) and are potent inotropic agents (25).

In the absence of a known structure it is particularly important to note certain criteria that must be met before a putative substance can be considered a serious candidate for a physiological regulator. Like all enzymes, Na^+-K^+-ATPase is readily inhibited by a very large number of substances. For example, the common fatty acids, linoleic and linolenic acid, are effective inhibitors (1, 29), though they exhibit a rather high inhibitory constant well beyond their physiological concentration (which, being in the millimolar range, is already several orders of magnitude greater than specific hormonal substances). Thus a believable physiologically relevant Na^+-K^+-ATPase inhibitor should have a very high binding affinity for the enzyme, at least within the order of magnitude of the cardiac glycosides ($\sim$2 nM).

If the function of the inhibitor is regulation of sodium-pump function, then reversibility of inhibition must be a cardinal criterion. Specificity for membrane Na^+-K^+-ATPase is also essential, since it would be cumbersome to regulate several enzymes at the same time. Finally, one would like to observe appropriate changes in inhibitor plasma concentration in response to relevant stimuli and to define a physiologically plausible mechanism of Na^+-K^+-ATPase inhibition. None of the putative substances put forward as candidates for the intrinsic Na^+-K^+-ATPase inhibitor meet all these criteria, and most have not been convincingly tested for one of them.

A low-molecular-weight nonpeptidic molecule can be extracted and partially purified from bovine hypothalamus, which has some of the characteristics and physiological properties of the cardiac glycosides (14). When small amounts of these partially purified extracts were applied to the serosal surface of the toad urinary bladder, a reversible nontoxic inhibition of active sodium transport across the membrane could be demonstrated. The inhibited sodium transport was accompanied by an increase in membrane resistance, indicating the inhibition was occurring through the active transport pathway and was not due to a toxic effect on the preparation. The factor was effective only from the serosal (circulatory) side of the membrane. When applied to the frog urinary bladder, a tissue that binds ouabain tightly, the factor inhibited binding of tritiated ouabain to its cellular receptor, the Na^+-K^+-ATPase. The Na^+-K^+-ATPase prepared from the renal medulla of the rabbit was then shown to be directly inhibited by the factor, and preliminary experiments showed that infusion of the factor into an isolated perfused rat kidney produced natriuresis. Thus this material had the characteristics of the putative natriuretic hormone and demonstrated biological properties similar to those of the cardiac glycosides.

The hypothalamic factor (HF) has been shown to be a low-molecular-weight nonpeptidic substance, since it elutes in the included volume on a Sephadex G-25 column and is resistant to acid hydrolysis (14). Activity is lost after ashing or base hydrolysis. The molecule appears to act as a zwitterion. At acid pH it behaves as a weak base and can be absorbed and eluted from strong cation-exchange resins (14). At neutral pH it appears to be anionic by its retention on anionic resins. The anionic behavior may be due to the presence of a carboxylic acid group, since the biological activity is lost after methylation by diazomethane and can be restored by gentle acid hydrolysis, as would be expected for a methyl ester. Complete characterization of the molecule with mass spectroscopy is in progress.

Endogenous factors that inhibit Na^+-K^+-ATPase activity or compete with ouabain for binding to the sodium pump have in general not been characterized with regard to the mechanism(s) of inhibition of enzyme activity or sodium transport; whether they are biochemically competent to assume a role in normal physiology has not been addressed. Using more highly purified hypothalamic factor, we designed experiments to determine affinity, reversibility, substrate specificity, and whether this factor demonstrates a physiologically plausible mechanism of Na^+-K^+-ATPase inhibition.

EXPERIMENTAL METHODS

The low-molecular-weight acid-stable HF was extracted, partially purified, and concentrated as previously described (4, 13). One unit of HF activity is defined arbitrarily as the amount of the inhibitor producing a 50% inhibition of enzyme activity under standard assay conditions in a coupled-enzyme assay after a 30-min preincubation at 37°C (13). This method links the hydrolysis of ATP to a regenerating system in which pyruvate kinase catalyzes the conversion of phospho*enol*pyruvate to pyruvate with the consequent reconversion of the ADP produced by ATP hydrolysis to ATP. This maintains ATP concentrations constant and prevents the accumulation of ADP, which is an ATPase inhibitor. The reaction is monitored by conversion of pyruvate to lactate, catalyzed by lactate dehydrogenase, which converts NADH to NAD^+. The latter is a chromophore, the concentration of which can be followed in a spectrophotometer; its degradation is stoichiometrically linked to the hydrolysis of ATP.

The Na^+-K^+-ATPase was purified from dog kidney by the procedure of Jorgensen (17) and stored frozen at $-70°C$. The specific ATPase activity measured in the coupled assay was 14–20 $\mu mol \cdot mg^{-1} \cdot min^{-1}$ at 37°C and was 98% ouabain inhibitable.

The Ca^{2+}-ATPase was isolated from rabbit hind and back muscle by the procedure of MacLennan (20), and Ca^{2+}-ATPase activity was measured in the coupled assay with 40 mM N-2-hydroxyethylpiperazine-N'-2-ethanesulfonic acid (HEPES), 2 mM ATP, 100 mM KCl, 5 mM $MgSO_4$, 0.4 mM ethylene glycol-bis(β-aminoethylether)-N,N'-tetraacetic acid (EGTA), 0.41 mM $CaCl_2$, and 1 mM ouabain.

Measurement of p-nitrophenylphosphatase (pNPPase) activity (initial velocity) and labeling with fluorescein-5′-isothiocyanate (FITC) was carried out as previously described (5). The stoichiometry of FITC labeling ranged from 2 to 3 nmol/mg protein. Fluorescence of FITC-labeled enzyme was measured on a spectrofluorometer with excitation wavelength 495 nm, emission at 520 nm.

Inside-out vesicles were prepared from fresh human erythrocytes by the method of Steck and Kant (28). The vesicles obtained were 80–90% inside out, as judged by the ratio of acetylcholinesterase activity in the presence and absence of detergent. The Na^+-K^+-ATPase activity of inside-out vesicles was determined by measuring strophanthidin-sensitive ouabain-resistant ATPase activity in the coupled assay in the presence of 1 μM valinomycin, 5 μg/ml monensin, 1 μg/ml fluorocyanocarbonylphenylhydrazone (FCCP), and 1 mM EGTA.

To study phosphorylation of Na^+-K^+-ATPase, 0.3 μg of dog kidney Na^+-K^+-ATPase in 20 μl of 20 mM Tris HCl, 5 mM $MgCl_2$, 2 mM norepinephrine, pH 7.4, was added to 20 μl of a solution of 20 mM $MgCl_2$, 100 μM H_3PO_4, 25 mM imidazole, 1 mM ethylenediaminetetraacetic acid (EDTA), pH 7.4, containing 30 μCi $[^{32}P]H_3PO_4$. The HF (2 units) or NaCl (0.55 M) was added to particular samples and incubated for the time indicated. Ouabain (1 mM) was added, and, after 10 min further incubation, 1.5 mg/ml bovine serum albumin were added; the reaction was stopped by addition of 10% trichloroacetic acid. After 15 min on ice the solution was centrifuged for 2 min in a microfuge; the pellet was washed with 5% trichloroacetic acid and resuspended by sonication into 100 μl of 1% sodium dodecyl sulfate. Aquasol (10 ml) was added and the sample counted for incorporation of ^{32}P.

The LLC-PK$_1$ cells were kept at 37°C, 5% CO_2, in Dulbecco's Modified Eagle Medium for 7–10 days until confluent and until domes appeared. Cells were dispersed prior to experiments by trypsinization. Medium was removed, the cells were washed once in zero Ca^{2+}/Mg^{2+} phosphate-buffered saline (PBS) at 37°C, and 4–5 ml of trypsin EDTA (zero Ca^{2+}/Mg^{2+}) were added to each culture dish (containing ~20 × 10^6 cells). After incubation at 37°C for 30 min, the cells were gently suspended by pipetting, placed in an equal volume of 10% fetal calf serum in complete PBS at 37°C, spun, and the supernatant aspirated. After two washes in complete PBS, the cells were resuspended as needed for individual experiments and kept at 37°C in a CO_2 incubator.

Pump activity was measured as ouabain-sensitive $^{86}Rb^+$ influx (J_{Rb}) into the LLC-PK$_1$ cells (13b); 5–10 × 10^6 cells were incubated in 100 mM NaCl, 5 mM KCl, 1 mM MgSO$_4$·7H$_2$O, 1.8 mM CaCl$_2$·2H$_2$O, 10 mM glucose, 25 mM HEPES, pH 7.4 for varying times with HF (20 U/ml) or ouabain (0.5 mM) and then cooled to create conditions for maximal pump activation. Cells were removed from the cold, placed at 37°C, and $^{86}Rb^+$ was added to make 0.012 μCi/μl in each tube. At the end of 10 min, 750 μl of cold buffer were added to the cell suspensions, 250 μl of 1:1 silicone:pthalate oil were layered over, the tubes were spun in a microfuge (10,000 g) for 2 min, and the unbound counts were removed by aspirating the upper layer (buffer) and most of the oil layer. The cell pellets were counted for γ-emission. Trapped counts in the pellet were <1%, as judged by ^{14}C inulin. Uptake in the presence of 0.5 mM ouabain was subtracted to determine ouabain-sensitive J_{Rb}. In some experiments cells were washed twice in cold buffer after the incubation with HF or ouabain, with subsequent addition of the $^{86}Rb^+$ to run the flux (washout experiments).

INHIBITION OF PURIFIED RENAL NA$^+$-K$^+$-ATPASE BY HYPOTHALAMIC FACTOR

Figure 1 shows the inhibition of Na$^+$-K$^+$-ATPase by HF with the use of the coupled-enzyme assay. Nearly complete inhibition can be demonstrated. Studies of the ligand requirements for binding to the purified enzyme indicated that magnesium is required for maximal inhibition by HF and that binding is diminished when sodium is present in the incubation mixture (13). To determine whether inhibition was reversible, the purified renal Na$^+$-K$^+$-ATPase was treated with HF in the presence of magnesium and then incubated with NaCl and EDTA. Assay of aliquots of this mixture over the next 2 h showed a reactivation of enzyme activity to the level seen when binding is done in the presence of NaCl and EDTA, with a half time of 1 h (Fig. 2). The effects of HF on the enzyme are thus reversible and not due to the effects of oxidizing agents or irreversible catalytic actions on the enzyme. These results are consistent with the finding of reversible inhibition of active sodium transport in toad urinary bladder (14).

HIGH-AFFINITY INHIBITION OF PURIFIED NA$^+$-K$^+$-ATPASE

Although HF has not been purified to homogeneity, it is possible to determine its affinity constant for the enzyme if the assumption is allowed that there is only one binding site per Na$^+$-K$^+$-ATPase molecule. The basis of this calculation is that when enzyme concentration exceeds inhibitor concentration, complete inhibition is not possible. Fifty-percent inhibition occurs

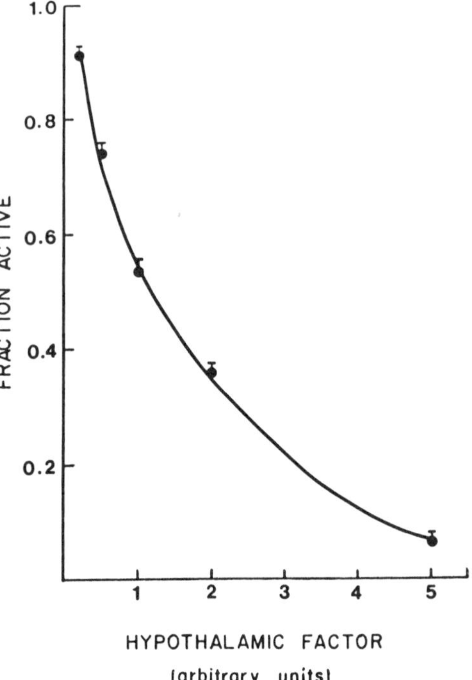

FIG. 1. Inhibition of purified Na$^+$-K$^+$-ATPase by increasing concentrations of hypothalamic factor (HF) as measured in the coupled-enzyme assay. After a 30-min incubation at 37°C, reaction mixtures were cooled on ice, diluted into assay buffer, and rate of residual Na$^+$-K$^+$-ATPase activity was determined spectrophotometrically. Fraction of enzyme remaining active was calculated by dividing initial velocity of HF samples by initial velocity of control samples. Data are means ± SE with $n \geqq 4$ at each inhibitor level (n, number of experiments). [Adapted from Haupert et al. (13).]

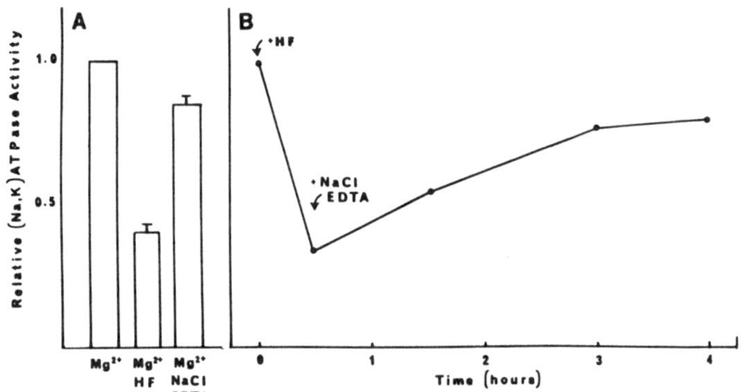

FIG. 2. A: inhibition of Na$^+$-K$^+$-ATPase activity by hypothalamic factor (HF). Purified dog kidney Na$^+$-K$^+$-ATPase was incubated at 0.1 mg/ml with HF (0.4 U/µg enzyme) in 20 mM Tris HCl, 5 mM MgCl$_2$, and 2 mM norepinephrine, pH 7.4, with or without 625 mM NaCl, and 7.5 mM ethylenediaminetetraacetic acid (EDTA) for 30 min at 37°C. Before and after incubation, 10-µl aliquots were withdrawn and assayed by the coupled assay. Values given as fraction of original activity. B: reactivation of HF-inhibited Na$^+$-K$^+$-ATPase activity. Dog kidney Na$^+$-K$^+$-ATPase was incubated as in A with HF added at time 0 and 625 mM NaCl and 7.5 mM EDTA added at time 0.5 h. Incubation was at 37°C; 10-µl aliquots were withdrawn at intervals to assay ATPase activity. Values given as fraction of control enzyme incubated without HF. [From Haupert et al. (13).]

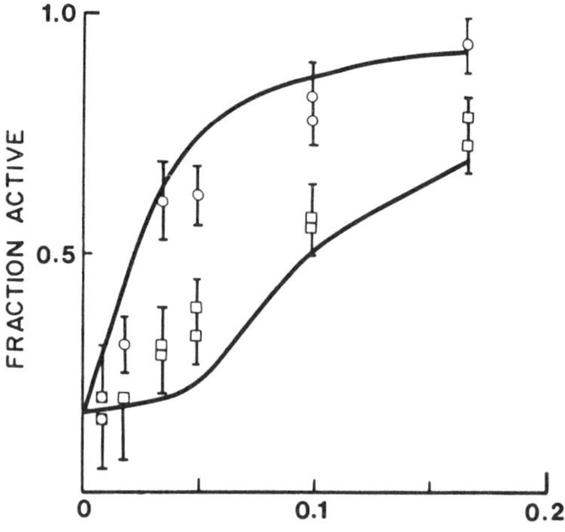

FIG. 3. Fraction of enzyme remaining active as measured in coupled assay after 30-min exposure of 1 (○) and 4 (□) U of hypothalamic factor (HF) to increasing concentrations of purified dog kidney Na^+-K^+-ATPase (2 separate determinations at each point). Incubations were carried out at 37°C in 50 μl of 20 mM Tris HCl, pH 7.4, containing 5 mM $MgCl_2$. Enzyme amounts are expressed as increasing concentrations of ouabain-binding sites where preparation of purified canine kidney enzyme contains 2.5 ± 0.5 nmol sites per milligram protein. Fraction of active enzyme at equilibrium may be expressed

$$\text{fraction active} = [E]/[E_t] = (K_i[E \cdot I])/([E_t][I_f]) \tag{1}$$

where [E] is the concentration of active enzyme, $[E_t]$ is the total concentration of enzyme, $[I_f]$ is the concentration of free HF, $[E \cdot I]$ is the concentration of inhibited enzyme, and K_i is the dissociation constant for the $E \cdot I$ complex. The relationship between total concentration of inhibitor $[I_t]$, $[E_t]$, and fraction of active enzyme molecules is

$$\text{fraction active} = (-A + \sqrt{A^2 + 4K_i[E_t]}/2[E_t]) \tag{2}$$

where $A = [I_t] + K_i - [E_t]$. Data at 2 different inhibitor concentrations were simultaneously fitted to *Equation 2* with a nonlinear least-squares computer program that permitted calculation of K_i and $[I_t]$. Two solid lines were drawn with K_i = 1.4 nM and $[I_t]$ = 15 nM and 60 nM, assuming 85% inhibition at low enzyme concentration. Fraction of enzyme remaining active was calculated by dividing initial velocity of HF samples by initial velocity of control samples. [From Haupert et al. (13).]

when enzyme concentration is approximately twice inhibitor concentration. This relationship is shown in Figure 3, where inhibitor concentration is fixed at 1 or 4 U and increasing concentrations of enzyme are added. The effect of the inhibitor is clearly titrated away by the enzyme and more readily at the lower inhibitor concentrations. If this were a low-affinity inhibitor, present in a high multiple of the concentration of the enzyme, it would be impossible to titrate the effect in this manner. The shape of the curve is consistent with a simple one-to-one inhibitor-enzyme interaction. A nonlinear least-squares program was used to fit data from the experiment at both concentrations to *Equation 2* in the legend of Figure 3. The result was K_i = 1.4 nM, where K_i is the dissociation constant. An alternative method for estimating the K_i is from the ratio of the reactivation rate constant to the inactivation rate constant. When this calculation was made the result was the same: $K_i = 1.4$ nM (13). Thus HF is a potent inhibitor of the Na^+-K^+-ATPase, with a binding affinity approximately two times greater than that of ouabain (24) and approximately six times greater than that of vanadate (18).

INHIBITION FROM THE EXTRACELLULAR SURFACE

Because HF inhibits cation transport in intact human erythrocytes (4), it was of interest to determine whether, like ouabain, this effect resulted from binding to the extracellular surface of the cell. As shown in Table 1, HF has little effect on Na^+-K^+-ATPase activity of inside-out erythrocyte vesicles but almost completely inhibits the Na^+-K^+-ATPase of detergent-permeabilized membranes. The Na^+-K^+-ATPase activity of intact vesicles was defined as that Na^+-K^+-ATPase activity that is resistant to ouabain (which does not permeate vesicles) but sensitive to strophanthidin (which is sufficiently hydrophobic to permeate the vesicles). Thus HF inhibits Na^+-K^+-ATPase activity only from the extracellular surface, again consistent with findings in the toad urinary bladder (14). An action from the extracellular surface is consistent with the concept of a circulating regulator of the sodium pump.

EFFECTS ON CONFORMATIONAL STATES AND PARTIAL REACTIONS OF NA^+-K^+-ATPASE

The Na^+-K^+-ATPase is believed to exist in two conformational states, E_1 and E_2, and the cycling of the enzyme between these two as ATP is hydrolyzed is felt to be required for transmembrane transport of sodium and potassium ions through the sodium pump (3). Sodium stabilizes the E_1 conformation and potassium stabilizes the E_2 state. These conformations can be readily distinguished by monitoring the fluorescence of FITC-labeled enzyme (19). In the absence of monovalent cations, the fluorescence of FITC-labeled enzyme that had been incubated with HF is similar to that of control enzyme (Table 2). The addition of 20 mM KCl to either control or HF-treated enzyme caused only a slight decrease in fluorescence, indicating that in the Tris buffer both

TABLE 1. *ATPase activity of inside-out vesicles*

	ATPase Activity, $nmol \cdot mg^{-1} \cdot min^{-1}$		
	Total	Strophanthidin sensitive	Strophanthidin resistant
IOV	3.8	1.1	2.7
IOV + HF	4.2	0.9	3.3
IOV + NP40	3.6	1.7	1.9
IOV + NP40 + HF	2.4	0.1	2.3

IOV, inside-out vesicles; HF, hypothalamic factor; NP40, Nonidet P-40. Error in data was ±15% (triplicate determinations). [Adapted from Haupert et al. (13a).]

TABLE 2. *Fluorescence of fluorescein-5′-isothiocyanate–labeled Na⁺-K⁺-ATPase*

	Control	+HF
20 mM Tris-Cl	1.00*	1.04
+20 mM KCl	0.95	0.98
+250 mM NaCl	1.30	1.04
+250 mM choline-Cl	1.00	1.01

Error in data was ±2%. HF, hypothalamic factor.   * Relative fluorescence units. [Adapted from Haupert et al. (13a).]

TABLE 3. *Effect of HF on p-nitrophenylphosphate–hydrolysis activity of Na⁺-K⁺-ATPase*

	pNPPase, μmol·mg^{-1}·min^{-1}	
	Enzyme	FITC-labeled enzyme*
Control	0.95	0.54
+HF	0.06†	0.09
+NaCl‡	0.03	0.06

Error in data was ±5%. HF, hypothalamic factor. FITC, fluorescein-5′-isothiocyanate. * Na⁺-K⁺-ATPase activity of FITC-labeled enzyme was 5% of activity of unmodified enzyme.   † Under identical conditions, HF caused 95% inhibition of Na⁺-K⁺-ATPase activity.   ‡ 0.5 M NaCl was added to pNPPase assay.   [Adapted from Haupert et al. (13a).]

enzymes were predominantly in the E_2 form. The addition of 250 mM NaCl reversed the effect of KCl on the control enzyme and caused a 30% further increase in fluorescence within 30 s. However, NaCl had only a slight effect on the HF-treated enzyme, causing a return to its original fluorescence intensity within 30 s but with no further change observed over the next 5 min. Choline-Cl (250 mM) had no effect on FITC fluorescence, suggesting that the changes observed were not merely due to an ionic strength effect. In this property, HF's mechanism is similar to that of ouabain.

Whereas ATP hydrolysis requires a transition between the E_1 and the E_2 states of Na⁺-K⁺-ATPase (fixing the enzyme in the E_2 state inhibits its action on ATP), the pseudosubstrate, p-nitrophenylphosphate (pNPP), may be hydrolyzed by the enzyme when maintained in its E_2 conformation. Both ouabain and HF are able to inhibit this action of the enzyme (Table 3).

INHIBITION OF PHOSPHORYLATION OF ACTIVE-SITE ASPARTATE RESIDUE OF NA⁺-K⁺-ATPASE

Because HF blocks ouabain binding to the Na⁺-K⁺-ATPase (15), we investigated its ability to substitute for ouabain in supporting phosphorylation of the active-site aspartate residue by inorganic phosphate and magnesium. As shown in Table 4, HF inhibits this ouabain-supported "back-door" phosphorylation of the Na⁺-K⁺-ATPase. Phosphorylation was decreased only when HF was allowed to equilibrate with the enzyme before the addition of ouabain.

TABLE 4. *Phosphorylation of Na^+-K^+-ATPase by $[^{32}P]H_3PO_4$*

Conditions	^{32}P Bound, nmol/mg
Ouabain, 10 min	1.2 ± 0.1
Ouabain + HF, 10 min	1.3 ± 0.1
HF (30 min) then ouabain + HF, 10 min	0.04 ± 0.1
HF, 40 min	0.0 ± 0.1
Ouabain, 40 min	1.2 ± 0.11

HF, hypothalamic factor. [Adapted from Haupert et al. (13a).]

TABLE 5. *Effect of hypothalamic factor on various membrane ATPases*

	ATPase Activity, $nmol \cdot mg^{-1} \cdot min^{-1}$			Inhibition, %
	Control	+HF, 0 min	+HF, 30 min	
Erythrocyte membrane				
Na^+-K^+-ATPase	10.0 ± 1.5*	10.0 ± 1.5	3.1 ± 1	70
Mg^+-ATPase	7.5 ± 1*	7.5 ± 1	6.6 ± 1	12
Ca^{2+}-ATPase	8.3 ± 1*	8.3 ± 1	8.4 ± 1	−1
Sarcoplasmic reticulum				
Ca^{2+}-ATPase	2,400*	2,400	864	64
Ca^{2+}-ATPase†	2,400*	2,400	1,080	55

* Activities changed <10% during 30-min incubation in buffer without hypothalamic factor (HF). † Preincubation buffer also contained 0.1 mM $CaCl_2$. [Adapted from Carilli et al. (4).]

This result is expected in view of the slow rate of HF binding to and release from the enzyme (13) and the high concentration of ouabain used (1 mM). The time dependence of the inhibition also makes it improbable that a low-affinity contaminant is affecting the back-door phosphorylation. In the absence of ouabain, HF did not stabilize back-door phosphorylation. Thus, although HF stabilizes an E_2-like conformation, it does not, unlike ouabain, stabilize the E_2-P bond and it prevents ouabain from stabilizing this bond.

SPECIFICITY OF HYPOTHALAMIC FACTOR INHIBITION

The effect of HF on erythrocyte membrane ATPase activities indicates a specificity for the Na^+-K^+-ATPase. The erythrocyte Mg^{2+}-ATPase and Ca^{2+}-ATPase were unaffected in membranes in which the Na^+-K^+-ATPase was inhibited by 75% (Table 5). However, the Ca^{2+}-ATPase of sarcoplasmic reticulum was inhibited by HF with a concentration dependence similar to that found for purified dog kidney Na^+-K^+-ATPase. Thus, although HF has a preference for inhibition of the Na^+-K^+ pump over other plasma membrane transport systems and ATPases, it also inhibits sarcoplasmic reticulum Ca^{2+}-ATPase.

REGULATION OF SODIUM-PUMP ACTIVITY IN INTACT CELLS

As shown in Figure 2, dissociation of HF from purified membrane preparations showed relatively slow off rates (off rates = 60 min). Since HF may be

TABLE 6. *Effect of hypothalamic factor and ouabain on ^{86}Rb influx in LLC-PK$_1$ cells*

	n	^{86}Rb Influx, μmol$\cdot$mg^{-1} DNA$\cdot$min^{-1}	P vs. Control
Control		15.2 $\pm$ 1.11	
+HF, 10 min	9	10.2 $\pm$ 1.34 (−33%)	<0.01
+HF, 60 min	9	0.61 $\pm$ 0.02 (−96%)	
+HF, 60 min + washout	8	30.5 $\pm$ 1.44 (+100%)	<0.001
+Ouabain, 60 min	2	2.8 (−81.6%)	
+Ouabain, 60 min + washout	2	3.2 (−78.6%)	

Data for hypothalamic factor (HF) are ouabain-sensitive ^{86}Rb influx; data for ouabain are total ^{86}Rb influx. n, Number of experiments.

a natriuretic hormone in vivo, binding and dissociation characteristics to the sodium pump were tested in LLC-PK$_1$ cells to assess physiological relevance (13b). These cells are an established line of renal tubular epithelial cells in which 80–90% of potassium transport occurs through the Na$^+$-K$^+$-ATPase. Pump activity was measured as ouabain-sensitive J_{Rb}, which serves as a tracer for potassium transport. As with membranes, a 60-min incubation with HF inhibited Na$^+$-K$^+$-ATPase activity (J_{Rb}) in LLC-PK$_1$ (Table 6). In contrast to membranes, no prior incubation with LLC-PK$_1$ was needed. Saturating HF produced an immediate 33% reduction of J_{Rb}. Removal of HF after 1 h of incubation showed rapid reversal of inhibition and provoked a 100% stimulation of J_{Rb}. Ouabain did not show this rapid dissociation of binding after washout (Table 6).

CONCLUSIONS

Although there has been a great deal of effort in many laboratories to identify and characterize a plasma, urinary, or tissue inhibitor of Na$^+$-K$^+$-ATPase, in general these substances have not been characterized with regard to the mechanism(s) of inhibition of enzyme activity or sodium transport, and the question of whether they are biochemically competent to assume a role in normal physiology has not been addressed. For a "new" natural compound to be presumed biologically relevant requires ultimately meeting a variety of stringent criteria. Central among these are the issues of affinity, reversibility, and specificity for substances felt to be regulatory in nature. In addition it is important to explore whether this factor(s) demonstrates a physiologically plausible mechanism of inhibition of the Na$^+$-K$^+$-ATPase.

I have recently addressed these issues with regard to the endogenous sodium-transport inhibitor extractable from bovine hypothalamus. The HF is both a high-affinity and reversible inhibitor of purified Na$^+$-K$^+$-ATPase in vitro (Figs. 2, 3). In addition, with regard to the plasma membrane, HF demonstrates specificity for the Na$^+$-K$^+$-ATPase, since at concentrations that inhibit Na$^+$-K$^+$-ATPase activity by 75%, Mg^{2+}- and Ca^{2+}-ATPase activities are not affected by HF (see Table 5). However, the Ca^{2+}-ATPase of sarcoplasmic reticulum was significantly inhibited. This may not be surprising in view of the structural homology between this enzyme and the Na^+-K^+-ATPase (26). Furthermore it may not be physiologically relevant, since HF has been shown to act only from the serosal surface in transporting epithelia (14) and only from the extracellular surface in the human erythrocyte (see Table 1). Thus the evidence is that HF does not penetrate the cell membrane and any potential activity on sarcoplasmic Ca^{2+}-ATPase may not be demonstrable in intact cells.

The mechanism of inhibition of the purified Na^+-K^+-ATPase by HF has been characterized and these activities have been compared with those of the cardiac glycoside, ouabain. Like ouabain, HF inhibits ion flux only from the extracellular side of the cell. This is important since a circulating inhibitor of Na^+-K^+-ATPase might explain certain effects associated with experimental (10) and human essential (11) hypertension and natriuretic effects associated with extracellular fluid volume expansion (14). Also like ouabain, HF inhibits one of the partial reactions of the Na^+-K^+-ATPase, the hydrolysis of the pseudosubstrate pNPP (see Table 3), and stabilizes an E_2-like conformation of the purified enzyme, as judged by fluorescence from FITC labeling (see Table 2). The HF, however, has significantly different ligand requirements from ouabain for binding to the Na^+-K^+-ATPase (13). Furthermore, unlike ouabain, HF does not support phosphorylation of the Na^+-K^+-ATPase from inorganic phosphate and magnesium and in fact blocks ouabain from supporting this back-door phosphorylation. This finding is consistent with the previous observation that phosphate partially protects the enzyme from HF inhibition (13).

Thus, although there are clear similarities between ouabain and HF in their interactions with Na^+-K^+-ATPase and in certain physiological effects, unequivocal mechanistic differences can be demonstrated. The HF is a unique inhibitor that may readily be differentiated from both the cardiac glycosides and vanadate. The evidence suggests that HF may inhibit Na^+-K^+-ATPase activity by influencing the phosphate-binding site and may alter active sodium transport by preventing the cycling of the enzyme between the E_1 and E_2 conformations.

Because on and off rates for HF binding in membrane preparations were relatively slow (off rates = 60 min), it was of interest to determine whether binding reactions in intact cells would show a time frame more consistent with physiological regulation in vivo. Binding and dissociation characteristics were studied in cultured renal tubular epithelial cells, LLC-PK$_1$. In contrast to isolated membranes, saturating HF produced immediate inhibition of the sodium pump in the intact cells, and removal of HF after 1 h of incubation showed rapid dissociation of the inhibitor and an actual stimulation of pump activity. The studies of ^{3}H-ouabain binding ongoing in our laboratory show that the enhanced transport is due to an increase in pump velocity and not to recruitment of additional pump units into the cell membrane. This pump stimulation is probably due to the accumulation of intracellular sodium during the pump inhibition by HF. With regard to regulation, it is tempting to postulate that the rapid reversal of HF binding to intact epithelial cells may be due to a shift to an enzyme conformation (E_1) unfavorable for HF binding, produced by transient increased intracellular sodium (and perhaps ATP) concentrations, since the combination of these ligands is known to "pull" the enzyme into E_1 and has been shown to inhibit HF binding to the purified Na^+-K^+-ATPase in vitro (13). Ouabain does not show the rapid dissociation of binding after washout (Table 6). The HF would appear to behave more physiologically than ouabain in regulation of Na^+-K^+-ATPase activity in these cells. In any case, these preliminary studies show that HF acts on renal cells as a potent regulator of Na^+-K^+-ATPase with a time frame quite different from that found in isolated membranes and consistent with physiological relevance. These effects could play an important role in the transepithelial movement of cations in the kidney that would account for a natriuretic effect in vivo.

REFERENCES

1. BIDARD, J.-N., B. ROSSI, J.-F. RENAUD, AND M. LAZDUNSKI. A search for an "ouabain-like" substance from the electric organ of *Electrophorus electricus* which led to arachidonic acid and related fatty acids. *Biochim. Biophys. Acta* 769: 245–252, 1984.
2. BOURGOIGNIE, J. J., K. H. HWANG, E. IPAKCHI, AND N. S. BRICKER. The presence of a natriuretic factor in urine of patients with chronic uremia. The absence of the factor in nephrotic uremic patients. *J. Clin. Invest.* 53: 1559–1567, 1974.
3. CANTLEY, L. C. Structure and mechanism of the Na,K-ATPase. *Curr. Top. Bioenerg.* 11: 201–237, 1981.
4. CARILLI, C. T., M. BERNE, L. C. CANTLEY, AND G. T. HAUPERT, JR. Hypothalamic factor inhibits the (Na,K)ATPase from the extracellular surface. Mechanism of inhibition. *J. Biol. Chem.* 260: 1027–1031, 1985.
5. CARILLI, C. T., R. A. FARLEY, D. M. PERLMAN, AND L. C. CANTLEY. The active site structure of Na^+- and K^+-stimulated ATPase. Location of a specific fluorescein isothiocyanate reactive site. *J. Biol. Chem.* 257: 5601–5606, 1982.
6. EDMONDSON, R. P. S., R. D. THOMAS, P. J. HILTON, J. PATRICK, AND N. F. JONES. Abnormal leucocyte composition and sodium transport in essential hypertension. *Lancet* 1: 1003–1005, 1975.
7. FINE, L. G., J. J. BOURGOIGNIE, K. H. HWANG, AND N. S. BRICKER. On the influence of the natriuretic factor from patients with chronic uremia on the bioelectric properties and sodium transport of the isolated mammalian collecting tubule. *J. Clin. Invest.* 58: 590–597, 1976.
8. FLIER, J., M. W. EDWARDS, J. W. DALY, AND C. W. MYERS. Widespread occurrence in frogs and toads of skin compounds interacting with the ouabain site of Na^+,K^+-ATPase. *Science Wash. DC* 208: 503–505, 1980.
9. HADDY, F. J., AND H. W. OVERBECK. The role of humoral agents in volume expanded hypertension. *Life Sci.* 19: 935–947, 1976.
10. HADDY, F. J., M. B. PAMNANI, AND D. L. CLOUGH. The sodium-potassium pump in volume expanded hypertension. *Clin. Exp. Hypertens.* 1: 295–336, 1978.
11. HAMLYN, J. M., R. RINGEL, J. SCHAEFFER, P. D. LEVINSON, B. P. HAMILTON, A. A. KOWARSKI, AND M. P. BLAUSTEIN. A circulating inhibitor of $(Na^+ + K^+)$ATPase associated with essential hypertension. *Nature Lond.* 300: 650–652, 1982.
12. HAUPERT, G. T., JR. Endogenous glycoside-like substances. In: *Current Topics in Membranes and Transport*, edited by J. F. Hoffmann and B. Forbush. New York: Academic, 1983, vol. 19, p. 843–855.
13. HAUPERT, G. T., JR., C. T. CARILLI, AND L. C. CANTLEY. Hypothalamic sodium-transport inhibitor is a high-affinity reversible inhibitor of Na^+-K^+-ATPase. *Am. J. Physiol.* 247 (*Renal Fluid Electrolyte Physiol.* 16): F919–F924, 1984.
13a.HAUPERT, G. T., JR., C. T. CARILLI, AND L. C. CANTLEY. Hypothalamic Na^+-transport

inhibitor: mechanism of inhibition. In: *The Sodium Pump*, edited by I. Glynn and C. Ellory. Cambridge, UK: Company of Biologists, 1985, p. 641–647.

13b.HAUPERT, G. T., JR., E. CHEN, S. RAY, AND H. F. CANTIELLO. Hypothalamic factor regulates sodium pump activity in cultured renal tubular epithelial cells. *Ann. NY Acad. Sci.* In press.

14. HAUPERT, G. T., JR., AND J. M. SANCHO. Sodium transport inhibitor from bovine hypothalamus. *Proc. Natl. Acad. Sci. USA* 76: 4658–4660, 1979.

15. HILLYARD, S. D., E. LU, AND H. C. GONICK. Further characterization of the natriuretic factor derived from kidney tissue of volume-expanded rats. Effects on short-circuit current and sodium-potassium-adenosine triphosphatase activity. *Circ. Res.* 38: 250–255, 1976.

16. HUGHES, J., T. W. SMITH, H. W. KOSTERLITZ, L. A. FOTHERGILL, B. A. MORGAN, AND H. R. MORRIS. Identification of two related pentapeptides from the brain with potent opiate agonist activity. *Nature Lond.* 258: 577–579, 1975.

17. JORGENSEN, P. L. Purification and characterization of $(Na^+ + K^+)$-ATPase. 3. Purification from the outer medulla of mammalian kidney after selective removal of membrane components by sodium dodecylsulphate. *Biochim. Biophys. Acta* 356: 36–52, 1974.

18. JOSEPHSON, L., AND L. C. CANTLEY, JR. Isolation of a potent (Na^+-K^+)ATPase inhibitor from striated muscle. *Biochemistry* 16: 4572–4578, 1977.

19. KARLISH, S. J., L. A. BEAUGÉ, AND I. M. GLYNN. Vanadate inhibits $(Na^+ + K^+)$ATPase by blocking a conformational change of the unphosphorylated form. *Nature Lond.* 282: 333–335, 1979.

20. MACLENNAN, D. H. Purification and properties of an adenosine triphosphatase from sarcoplasmic reticulum. *J. Biol. Chem.* 245: 4508–4518, 1970.

21. OVERBECK, H. W., M. B. PAMNANI, T. AKERA, T. M. BRODY, AND F. J. HADDY. Depressed function of a ouabain-sensitive sodium-potassium pump in blood vessels from renal hypertensive dogs. *Circ. Res.* 38, Suppl. 2: 48–52, 1976.

22. POSTON, L., R. B. SEWELL, S. P. WILKINSON, P. J. RICHARDSON, R. WILLIAMS, E. M. CLARKSON, G. A. MACGREGOR, AND H. E. DE WARDENER. Evidence for a circulating sodium transport inhibitor in essential hypertension. *Br. Med. J.* 282: 847–849, 1981.

23. SCHMIDT, R. W., J. J. BOURGOIGNIE, AND N. S. BRICKER. On the adaptation in sodium excretion in chronic uremia. The effects of "proportional reduction" of sodium intake. *J. Clin. Invest.* 53: 1736–1741, 1974.

24. SCHWARTZ, A., K. WHITMER, G. GRUPP, I. GRUPP, R. J. ADAMS, AND S. W. LEE. Mechanism of action of digitalis: is the Na,K-ATPase the pharmacological receptor? *Ann. NY Acad. Sci.* 402: 253–271, 1982.

25. SHIMONI, Y., M. GOTSMAN, J. DEUTSCH, S. KACHALSKY, AND D. LICHTSTEIN. Endogenous ouabain-like compound increases heart muscle contractility. *Nature Lond.* 307: 369–371, 1984.

26. SHULL, G. E., A. SCHWARTZ, AND J. B. LINGREL. Amino-acid sequence of the catalytic subunit of the $(Na^+ + K^+)$ATPase deduced from a complementary DNA. *Nature Lond.* 316: 691–695, 1985.

27. SIMANTOV, R., AND S. H. SNYDER. Morphine-like peptides in mammalian brain: isolation, structure elucidation, and interactions with the opiate receptor. *Proc. Natl. Acad. Sci. USA* 73: 2515–2519, 1976.

28. STECK, T., AND J. KANT. Preparation of impermeable ghosts and inside-out vesicles from human erythrocyte membranes. *Methods Enzymol.* 31: 172–180, 1974.

29. TAMURA, M., H. KUWANO, T. KINOSHITA, AND T. INAGAMI. Identification of linoleic and oleic acids as endogenous Na^+,K^+-ATPase inhibitors from acute volume-expanded hog plasma. *J. Biol. Chem.* 260: 9672–9677, 1985.

30. WARDENER, H. E. DE, I. H. MILLS, W. F. CLAPHAM, AND C. J. HAYTER. Studies on the efferent mechanism of the sodium diuresis which follows the administration of intravenous saline in the dog. *Clin. Sci. Lond.* 21: 249–258, 1961.

31. WELT, L. G., J. R. SACHS, AND T. J. MANUS. An ion transport defect in erythrocytes from uremic patients. *Trans. Assoc. Am. Physicians* 77: 169–181, 1964.

14

Natriuretic Factors in Arterial Hypertension

FRANCIS J. HADDY AND MOTILAL B. PAMNANI

Department of Physiology, Uniformed Services University, Bethesda, Maryland

Evidence From Reduced Renal Mass–Saline Hypertension in the Rat
Literature Survey
Hypothesis
Conclusions

THE POSSIBLE ROLES OF NATRIURETIC FACTORS in arterial hypertension are addressed in this chapter. We suspect that natriuretic factors are most important in the low-renin forms of arterial hypertension, i.e., those forms with *1*) low plasma renin activity, *2*) relative insensitivity to angiotensin antagonists and converting enzyme inhibitors, *3*) relative sensitivity to dietary salt restriction and natriuretic-diuretic medication, and *4*) absolute or relative volume expansion. Typical examples of these forms of hypertension are, in humans, primary aldosteronism, renal parenchymal disease, and low-renin essential hypertension in black male patients; examples in animals are reduced renal mass–saline hypertension; one-kidney, one clip hypertension; and one-kidney, deoxycorticosterone acetate (DOCA), saline hypertension. In this chapter we present our reasons for suspecting important roles for natriuretic factors in low-renin hypertension. Only two natriuretic factors are considered: one (de Wardener) that operates by inhibiting the sodium pump and one of atrial origin (de Bold) that does not.

The evidence for important roles for these natriuretic factors in low-renin arterial hypertension is most complete for the rat with reduced renal mass–saline hypertension (5, 38, 39, 59, 62, 64). We therefore highlight this classic form of low-renin hypertension.

EVIDENCE FROM REDUCED RENAL MASS–SALINE
HYPERTENSION IN THE RAT

It has long been known that a certain percentage of common laboratory animals become hypertensive when their sodium chloride intake is increased (30). It is also known that this hypertension in the rat, dog, and monkey occurs more regularly, rapidly, and severely if renal function is first reduced (30). This finding has been particularly well documented in dogs and rats with 70–80% surgical reduction of renal mass (7, 16, 66, 90, 91); increased sodium intake now almost always produces a rapid and dramatic increase in arterial pressure. These rats with reduced renal mass on a high-salt intake are volume expanded with low plasma renin activity (39, 66, 90). If, however, the dietary sodium intake of subtotally nephrectomized rats is reduced in direct proportion to the decrease in glomerular filtration rate, the rats remain normotensive (16, 66, 91). In 1974 Schmidt et al. (73) showed that a serum fraction from dogs uremic because of 85% surgical reduction of renal mass contains a substance that causes natriuresis when injected into assay rats. The substance disappeared with dietary sodium restriction but the uremia did not. In that same year, Kramer and Gonick (46) showed that acute volume expansion inhibits renal Na^+- and K^+-activated ATPase (Na^+-K^+-ATPase), and in 1976 Hillyard et al. (34) showed that it also produces an agent in the kidney that inhibits Na^+-K^+-ATPase obtained from normal kidney. We then generated evidence for increased plasma levels of an inhibitor of the sodium pump in the vascular smooth muscle cells of rats with reduced renal mass–saline hypertension (38, 39, 62).

Our studies in rats with reduced renal mass–saline hypertension followed others in dogs with one-kidney, one wrap hypertension that revealed reduced ouabain-sensitive ^{86}Rb uptake (an index of sodium-pump activity) in the arteries and veins (57, 61, 62) and an agent in plasma that reduced ouabain-sensitive ^{86}Rb uptake when applied to the tail artery from a normal rat (61, 62). They also followed still others that revealed that the same is true for normal dogs and rats after acute volume expansion with saline (61). In the reduced renal mass–saline studies (5, 38, 39, 62), 70–80% of renal mass was removed surgically from a group of rats and the rats were then placed on a low-sodium diet (0.02%). Half drank distilled water; the other half drank a 1% solution of sodium chloride (saline). Those drinking distilled water remained normotensive, whereas those drinking saline rapidly became significantly hypertensive within one week and the pressure continued to increase at a slower rate over the next four weeks. Both were uremic, the normotensive animals slightly more than the hypertensive animals (blood urea nitrogen 49 and 38 mg%, creatinine 1.1 and 1.1 mg%, respectively, 5 wk after surgery). At various times after surgery, but particularly at the end of the fifth week, the animals were anesthetized with pentobarbital sodium. Their tail arteries and hearts were removed for measurement of ouabain-sensitive ^{86}Rb uptake and microsomal Na^+-K^+-ATPase activity, respectively; their blood was removed for bioassay of plasma for sodium-pump inhibitory activity. In this bioassay, boiled plasma supernatant from a hypertensive animal is applied to half of a tail artery from a normal animal while supernatant from a normotensive animal is applied to the other half. Ouabain-sensitive ^{86}Rb uptake is then measured in each half and the values compared. In a second bioassay, we used microelectrodes to measure membrane potentials of vascular smooth muscle cells in normal rat tail artery halves before and after application of plasma supernatant from hypertensive or normotensive rats. In some studies the animals had anteroventral third ventricle (AV3V) lesions or central sympathectomies (intraventricular 6-hydroxydopamine). In others, measurements were made after reversal of the hypertension by switching the drinking fluid from saline to water.

Relative to the normotensive animals, the hypertensive animals had

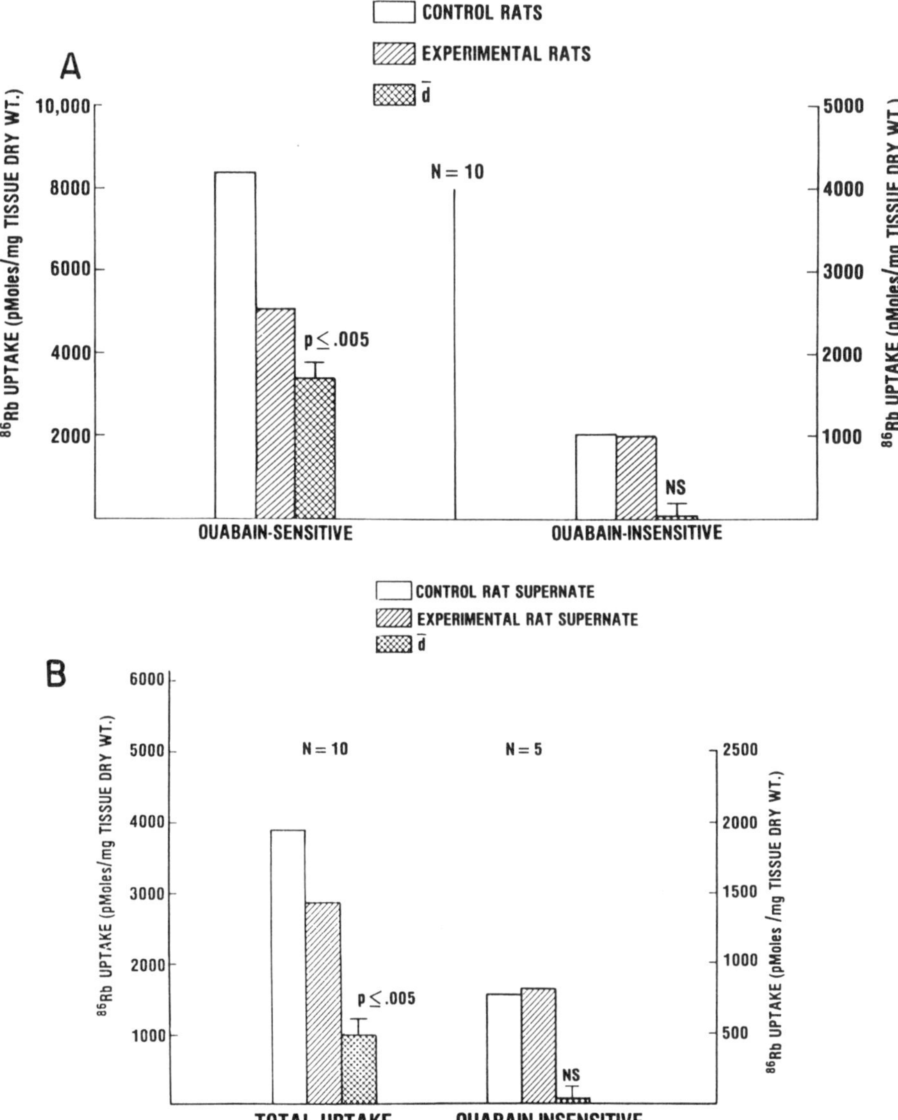

FIG. 1. A: ouabain-sensitive and ouabain-insensitive ^{86}Rb uptake by tail arteries from reduced renal mass, water-drinking, normotensive (control) and reduced renal mass, saline-drinking, hypertensive (experimental) rats. d̄, Mean difference between control and experimental rats. B: effects of supernatants of boiled plasma from hypertensive and normotensive rats on total and ouabain-insensitive uptake by tail arteries from normal rats. Two uptakes were measured in different tail arteries for lack of sufficient supernatant volume. [From Pamnani et al. (62), by permission of the American Heart Association, Inc.]

increased extracellular fluid volume (39), decreased plasma renin activity (39), increased plasma sodium-pump inhibitory activity [plasma supernatants reduced ouabain-sensitive ^{86}Rb uptake (Fig. 1B) and membrane potential in tail artery halves from normal animals (5, 38, 39, 62)], decreased cardiac microsomal Na^+-K^+-ATPase activity (6, 38, 39), and decreased tail artery sodium-potassium–pump activity (Fig. 1A) (even after in vitro chemical sympathectomy) (38, 39, 62). Appearance of the decreased pump activity was temporally associated with the development of the hypertension (39). The AV3V lesions and central sympathectomy prevented the appearance of 1) increased plasma sodium-pump inhibitory activity, 2) decreased vascular sodium-potassium–pump activity, and 3) increased blood pressure (38). Reversal of the hypertension by switching the drinking fluid from saline to water also reversed the changes in plasma sodium-pump inhibitory activity (38), vascular sodium-potassium–pump activity (38), and myocardial Na^+-K^+-ATPase activity (6).

Atrial extract does not inhibit the sodium pump. This was recognized in several laboratories very quickly after de Bold et al. (9) discovered its natriuretic properties. In 1981 we extracted rat atria and ventricles in cold phosphate-buffered saline or distilled water and confirmed that atrial extract does indeed have potent natriuretic and diuretic properties in bioassay rats, whereas ventricular extract is without effect (50, 60). We then tested the effects of the two extracts on Na^+-K^+-ATPase derived from heart and also from renal cortex and found, like Thibault et al. (81), that atrial extract does not inhibit Na^+-K^+-ATPase activity relative to ventricular extract. We incubated rat tail arteries in atrial and ventricular extracts and measured ouabain-sensitive ^{86}Rb uptake, an index of sodium-potassium–pump activity, and found no difference. We then exposed toad bladders to atrial and ventricular extracts and measured short-circuit current and found no difference in the antinatriferic activities. Thus, even though atrial extract is natriuretic and ventricular extract is not, we found no differences in their effects on Na^+-K^+-ATPase, the sodium-potassium pump, and short-circuit current. These findings indicated that atrial natriuretic factor (ANF) is not natriuretic by virtue of Na^+-K^+-ATPase inhibition. Because the humoral sodium-pump inhibitor found in volume-expanded states does inhibit Na^+-K^+-ATPase and the sodium-potassium pump, we concluded that the two agents are not one and the same.

Atrial extract does have potent natriuretic and diuretic properties, however. We infused the extracts into bioassay rats and found, like others, that the atrial extract produces a prompt massive transient natriuresis and diuresis, whereas the ventricular extract is essentially without effect. We were not impressed with its hemodynamic activity. For example, relative to ventricular extract, 10 min of intravenous infusion of the atrial extract into the bilaterally nephrectomized, hexamethonium-treated or bilaterally nephrectomized, autonomically blocked (phentolamine, propranol, and atropine) rat had no effect, except transiently, on blood pressure (60, 63).

More recently we have bioassayed atrial extracts from hypertensive rats for natriuretic and diuretic activity. Among them were rats with reduced renal mass–saline hypertension (59). Intravenous administration of atrial extract prepared from rats with four weeks of reduced renal mass–saline hypertension produced more natriuresis and diuresis in the bioassay rats than did atrial extract from normotensive control animals (water-drinking rats with reduced renal mass) (59). This difference was not present three days after reversal of the hypertension by switching the drinking fluid from saline to water. These findings were similar to those in the Dahl salt-sensitive (S) rat (49). Here atrial extracts were prepared from Dahl S rats and Dahl salt-resistant (R) rats receiving high- and low-salt diets. Atrial extracts from S rats produced more diuresis and natriuresis than extracts from R rats, regardless of the salt intake, and extracts from S rats receiving a high-salt diet produced more diuresis and natriuresis than extracts from S rats receiving a low-salt diet. Furthermore, as in the study of Hirata et al. (35), the kidney of the normotensive Dahl S rat was less sensitive than the kidney of the Dahl R rat to atrial extract prepared from a normal rat.

We wondered whether ANF, through its potent diuretic and natriuretic properties, plays a compensatory role, preventing excessive elevation of blood pressure, in rats with reduced renal mass–saline hypertension. We therefore blocked the in vivo action of ANF in rats with 60% reduction (slightly less than our usual 70–80% reduction) in renal mass to evaluate the effect on blood pressure (64). Blockade was accomplished with anti-ANF antibody prepared in rabbits against the COOH-terminal heptapeptide of atriopeptin III (AP III). We used rats with 60% reduction in renal mass because these animals remain normotensive on the sodium-deficient diet plus 1% saline, but any slight further reduction in renal mass induces hypertension. Following the 60% reduction in renal mass, all animals consumed a sodium-deficient diet (0.02% sodium) and drank a 1% solution of sodium chloride and remained normotensive. Four weeks later the animals were divided into two groups. One group was injected intraperitoneally daily with rabbit serum containing the antibody; the other group received normal rabbit serum. Blood pressure increased in the first group from 126 to 158 mmHg by the 12th day; after withdrawal of the antibody, blood pressure returned to control values in 5–6 days. Treatment and withdrawal of normal rabbit serum in the second group of rats had no effect on blood pressure. These studies show that in normotensive rats primed for hypertension with reduction in renal mass, ANF antibody raises blood pressure. They suggest that ANF modulates the development of hypertension in rats with reduced renal mass.

LITERATURE SURVEY

Tables 1 and 2 present conditions in which bioassay and/or radioimmunoassay for sodium-pump inhibitory activity and ANF have been reported to be abnormal. In the case of the sodium-pump inhibitor, certain conditions (acute volume expansion, increased dietary salt, chronic renal failure, essential hypertension) have been studied by many investigators (see refs. cited in 32, 33, and 82a). In the case of ANF, the conditions have not been reviewed. Indeed, many of the studies have only been reported in abstracts. All ANF studies known to the authors are therefore cited, but completeness is not claimed.

TABLE 1. *Normotensive conditions in which bioassay and radioimmunoassay for sodium-pump inhibitor and atrial natriuretic factor were abnormal*

Condition	Sodium-Pump Inhibitor		Atrial Natriuretic Factor	
	Plasma	Urine	Atrial tissue	Plasma
Acute volume expansion	↑ (82a)	↑ (82a)		↑ (4, 18, 20, 47, 65, 70, 78, 84, 87)
Immersion to neck	↑ (14)	↑ (14)		↑ (56)
Increased dietary salt	↑ (82a)	↑ (82a)	↓ (69)	↓ (68)
			↑ (49*, 67, 80a)	↑ (28, 36, 37, 75a, 80a)
Chronic hypoxia			↓ (52)	↑ (52)
Upright posture				↓ (36)
Pregnancy	↑ (83)			↑ (8)
Newborn	↑ (83)			
Chronic renal failure	↑ (82a)	↑ (82a)		↑ (75)
Bilateral ureteral ligation				↑ (19)
Cirrhosis	↓ (44)	↓ (17, 54)		↑ (23)
	↑ (74)			
Congestive heart failure			↓ (5a, 13)	↑ (40, 55, 75a, 82, 85)
Paroxysmal atrial tachycardia				↑ (43, 72, 82, 86, 88†)
Cardiac pacing				↑ (88†)
Right atrial distension				↑ (3, 12, 48, 58, 71)

Table is not all-inclusive. Numbers in parentheses are reference numbers. ↑, Increased; ↓, decreased.   *Dahl salt-sensitive rat.   †Coronary sinus plasma.

For the most part, the conditions listed in Tables 1 and 2 are associated with central volume expansion. In one condition, upright posture, the reverse is the case. The conditions associated with central volume expansion are also associated with increased plasma levels of both the sodium-pump inhibitor and ANF. The upright-posture condition is associated with a decreased plasma level of ANF. Immersion to the neck, which selectively increases central blood volume, increases the plasma level of both agents. Atrial distension, even in vitro (3, 12, 71), increases the plasma level of ANF.

In some cases the data are not uniform. In cirrhosis of the liver, one group of investigators reported increased plasma levels of the inhibitor (74) but another group (44) reported decreased levels; one group reported increased plasma levels of ANF (23) while another reported no change (75a). The variable data in cirrhosis have been discussed (15, 23). With increased dietary salt intake, five groups reported an increase in the plasma level of ANF while one group reported a decrease, and three groups reported an increase in the atrial level while one reported a decrease (Table 1). In the Okamoto spontaneously hypertensive rat (SHR), two groups reported an increase in the plasma level

TABLE 2. *Hypertensive conditions in which bioassay and radioimmunoassay for sodium-pump inhibitor and atrial natriuretic factor were abnormal*

Condition	Sodium-Pump Inhibitor		Atrial Natriuretic Factor	
	Plasma	Urine	Atrial tissue	Plasma
Primary aldosteronism	↑ (45)			
Renal failure	↑ (79)			
Pregnancy, amniotic fluid		↑ (25)		
Acromegaly	↑ (10)			
Essential, especially low renin	↑ (32, 33)			↑ (2)
Okamoto spontaneously hypertensive rat		↓ (89)	↓ (22, 27, 51, 53, 77)	↓ (51)
			↑ (69)	↑ (27, 53)
Dahl salt-sensitive rat, high-salt diet			↑ (35, 49, 69)	↑ (80a)
Reduced renal mass–saline, rat	↑ (38, 39, 62)		↑ (59)	
One-kidney, one clip, rat	↑ (62)		↓ (21, 22)	↑ (R. Garcia, personal communication)
Deoxycorticosterone, salt, rat	↑ (42, 76)*		↓ (41)† ↑ (1)†	↑ (41)
One-kidney, one wrapped, dog	↑ (61, 62)			
Mineralocorticoid (during development), two kidney				↑ (24‡, 26§)

Table is not all-inclusive. Numbers in parentheses are reference numbers. ↑, Increased; ↓, decreased. *One kidney. †Two kidney. ‡Dog. §Pig.

of ANF (27, 53), two reported no change (4, 65), and one reported a decrease (51); five reported decreased atrial levels but one reported increased atrial levels (Table 2). In reduced renal mass–saline hypertension, one group reported an increase in the atrial tissue level of ANF (59) while another reported no change (22). In DOCA-salt hypertension, opposite changes in atrial levels were reported by two groups (Table 2).

In the case of ANF, these apparent discrepancies may in part be related to differences in the antisera used to perform the radioimmunoassay. For example, Fried et al. (20) used two different antisera, one highly selective for 28–amino acid α-rat atrial natriuretic peptide (α-rANP) and the other having 100% cross-reactivity with 28–amino acid α-rANP but also reacting with other ANP species, to measure plasma natriuretic peptide levels in the rat during acute volume expansion. With the first antisera, the control level was lower and did not change with volume expansion; with the second antisera, the level increased fourfold within one minute of volume expansion. The apparent discrepancies may also be related to differences in the time of measurement. For example, R. Garcia (personal communication) found the atrial level of ANF decreased during the first two weeks after creation of one-kidney, one clip hypertension in the rat but normal thereafter. In SHR the atrial level is apparently reduced only in the adult animal; normal or elevated levels have been found in the young (27, 51, 69). Finally, the apparent discrepancies may be related to the method of measurement. For example, Ackermann and Irizawa (1) estimated atrial levels by bioassay and Kihara et al. (41) estimated them by radioimmunoassay and obtained opposite results after administration of DOCA and salt to the rat. Were they measuring the same variable? That is, does radioimmunoassay always reflect biological activity in atrial extracts? Tanaka and Inagami (80) consider this possibility in relation to their findings and those of Hirata et al. (35) in the Dahl S rat.

In seven conditions, both plasma and atrial tissue levels of ANF are available. These are *1*) increased dietary salt, *2*) chronic hypoxia, *3*) congestive heart failure, *4*) spontaneous hypertension, *5*) Dahl S, *6*) one-kidney, one clip hypertension, and *7*) DOCA-salt hypertension. Although the data are not uniform in all cases, in five of the seven conditions increased plasma levels are associated with decreased atrial levels (the exceptions are increased dietary salt in Table 1 and Dahl S in Table 2). Such findings suggest a reciprocal relationship between atrial and plasma levels. Apparently elevated atrial pressure can cause release in excess of synthesis, resulting in elevated plasma levels and decreased atrial levels. Several of the studies suggest, however, that with time synthesis catches up with release, resulting in elevated plasma levels and normal (one-kidney, one clip) or even elevated atrial levels (increased dietary salt, Dahl S, reduced renal mass–saline). Note that elevated atrial levels have been associated only with the chronic administration of salt.

Most of the conditions listed in Tables 1 and 2 have been reviewed previously in relation to the sodium-pump inhibitor (32, 33, 82a, 83). The notable exception is acromegaly. Devynck and Meyer (10) recently reported the ability of plasma extracts from six active and seven cured acromegalics to compete with [^{3}H]ouabain for binding to red cells from normal human subjects. The active acromegalic patients were characterized by an expanded plasma volume, elevated blood pressure, and a positive binding assay (the increased ability of the plasma extracts to displace [^{3}H]ouabain was more regular than in any other group of patients studied). The three abnormalities were not found in the seven cured patients. The uniformity of the increased activity in the plasma of the active acromegalic patients may be relevant to the source of the sodium-pump inhibitor.

Perhaps the major message in Tables 1 and 2 is that abnormally high plasma levels of both agents, sodium-pump inhibitor and ANF, are found in conditions characterized by volume expansion.

HYPOTHESIS

We here concentrate on the possible roles of the sodium-pump inhibitor and ANF in the genesis and maintenance of low-renin hypertension, based largely on our experience with reduced renal mass–saline hypertension and on the data in Tables 1 and 2. Previously we presented a hypothesis utilizing the sodium-pump inhibitor (29–32). Here we incorporate the ANF.

Our working hypothesis is that an inability to excrete sodium normally, due to genetic or acquired renal defects, leads to increased blood volume, particularly when sodium intake increases. The rise in pressure in the central circulation increases the release of a sodium-pump inhibitor that, through actions on cardiovascular muscle, leads to increased contractile activity and hence pressure. This, along with its actions on the renal tubule, tends to normalize volume via diuresis. The rise in pressure in the central circulation also increases the release of ANF, which also tends to reverse this sequence by increasing the ability of the kidney to excrete sodium and water. Thus our current thinking is that, in low-renin hypertension, the elevated pressure is generated by a sodium-pump inhibitor acting on heart and blood vessels and is compensated by pressure, sodium-pump inhibitor, and ANF acting on the kidney.

This hypothesis is best supported by data from the reduced renal mass–saline model of low-renin hypertension. In this model we demonstrated *1)* increased blood and extracellular fluid volumes; *2)* sodium-pump inhibition in blood vessels, which correlates temporally with the onset and offset of the hypertension; *3)* Na^+-K^+-ATPase inhibition in myocardial microsomes, which disappears on curing the hypertension; *4)* increased levels of a sodium-pump inhibitor in the plasma, which disappear on curing the hypertension; *5)* increased atrial tissue levels of ANF, which disappear on curing the hypertension; and *6)* the appearance of hypertension on administration of an antisera to ANF in rats with reduction in renal mass, which is just insufficient by itself to raise pressure.

The data in Table 1 show that increased blood volume, via atrial distension, leads to increased blood levels of ANF. Intravenous administration of ANP causes diuresis and decreased blood pressure in normal animals and humans. Thus it is difficult to explain low-renin volume-expanded hypertension via increased blood levels of ANF; i.e., it would be illogical to suggest that an excess of ANF causes hypertension. It seems more likely that an excess of ANF compensates increased volume and pressure.

A deficiency of ANF might raise pressure, but decreased blood levels have been reported in only one study of arterial hypertension (Table 2). In theory, ANF could generate hypertension, rather than compensate it, if some defect led to decreased blood levels or decreased responses to it. Blood pressure might increase both because of lack of a natriuretic hormone action (decreased production, decreased release, decreased renal response) or lack of a vasorelaxant action (decreased production, decreased release, decreased blood vessel response). However, blood levels have been reported to be increased in essential hypertension, in two of five studies in the SHR, in the Dahl S hypertensive rat, in one-kidney, one clip hypertension in the rat, during the development of mineralocorticoid hypertension in the dog and pig, and during the sustained phase of DOCA-salt hypertension in the rat (Table 2). Only one group, studying the SHR, reported decreased plasma levels. Atrial tissue levels have been reported to be decreased in the adult SHR, in the DOCA-salt hypertensive rat, and in the one-kidney, one clip hypertensive rat (Table 2). However,

Garcia et al. (21) speculate that the lower concentration of ANF in the atria of one-kidney, one clip rats reflects an increased release into the circulation, triggered by an increased circulatory volume and an increased intra-auricular pressure, and functions as a compensatory mechanism that prevents further increments in blood pressure and plasma volume.

Certain defects should speed the development of low-renin hypertension. For example, if the sodium-pump inhibitor is superimposed on vascular smooth muscle cells that are abnormally permeable to sodium, intracellular sodium concentration will rise more quickly and to higher levels, thereby exaggerating the hypertension. Deteriorating renal function or increased salt intake in the SHR might produce this combination. Kidneys that are hyporesponsive to ANF should also exaggerate the hypertension. This may occur in the Dahl S rat. Hirata et al. (35) showed that the hypertensive Dahl S rat has more extractable tissue ANF than the normotensive Dahl R rat (both on a high-salt diet) but that its kidneys are less responsive to exogenous ANF. Link et al. (49) confirmed these findings.

CONCLUSIONS

This chapter considers the possible roles of a sodium-pump inhibitor and ANF in arterial hypertension; data are used from the rat with reduced renal mass–saline hypertension and from the literature. Based on these data, including the data indicating that both agents are released by volume expansion, our view is that low-renin hypertension is in part generated by the sodium-pump inhibitor and that this hypertension is in part moderated by ANF. We suggest that the ANF system compensates for increased volume due to reduced renal function and/or increased salt intake and that in low-renin hypertension the compensation is not sufficient to return volume and pressure to normal. In this view the sodium-pump inhibitor is prohypertensive, via actions on blood vessels and heart, and ANF is antihypertensive, via actions on kidney and perhaps blood vessels.

REFERENCES

1. ACKERMANN, U., AND T. G. IRIZAWA. Synthesis and renal activity of rat atrial granules depend on extracellular volume. *Am. J. Physiol.* 247 (*Regulatory Integrative Comp. Physiol.* 16): R750–R752, 1984.
2. ARENDT, R. M., E. STANGL, AND J. ZÄHRINGER. Alpha-atrial natriuretic factor in human plasma: difference between normotensive and hypertensive patients (abstr.). *Circulation* 72, Suppl. III: III103, 1985.
3. BILDER, G. E., AND E. H. BLAINE. Release of atrial natriuretic factor with continuous and repetitive stretch (abstr.). *Federation Proc.* 45: 527, 1986.
4. BRAVO, E. L., M. KIHARA, K. NAKAO, N. MORII, A. SUGAWARA, M. KIHARA, H. IMURA, AND Y. YAMORI. Atrial natriuretic peptide: the regulatory role of volume and the sympathetic nervous system (abstr.). In: *Int. Symp. Rats Spontaneus Hypertension Related Studies, 5th, Kyoto, Japan, Oct. 20–22, 1985*, p. 154.
5. BRYANT, H. J., M. B. PAMNANI, D. R. HARDER, S. J. HUOT, AND F. J. HADDY. Vascular smooth muscle membrane potentials (Em) in rats with reduced renal mass (RRM)

hypertension: the influence of a ouabain-like humoral factor (abstr.). *Federation Proc.* 44: 1749, 1985.

5a. CHIMOSKEY, J. E., W. S. SPIELMAN, M. A. BRANDT, AND S. R. HEIDEMANN. Cardiac atria of BIO 14.6 hamsters are deficient in natriuretic factor. *Science Wash. DC* 223: 820–822, 1984.

6. CLOUGH, D. L., S. J. HUOT, M. B. PAMNANI, AND F. J. HADDY. Decreased myocardial Na⁺,K⁺-ATPase activity in rats with reduced renal mass-saline hypertension. *J. Hypertens.* 3: 583–589, 1985.

7. COLEMAN, T. G., AND A. C. GUYTON. Hypertension caused by salt loading in the dog. 3. Onset transients of cardiac output and other variables. *Circ. Res.* 25: 153–160, 1969.

8. CUSSON, J. R., J. GUTKOWSKA, E. REY, N. MICHON, M. BOUCHER, AND P. LAROCHELLE. Plasma concentration of atrial natriuretic factor in normal pregnancy (Letter to the editor). *N. Engl. J. Med.* 313: 1230–1231, 1985.

9. DE BOLD, A. J., H. B. BORENSTEIN, A. T. VERESS, AND H. A. SONNENBERG. A rapid and potent natriuretic response to intravenous injection of atrial myocardial extract in rats. *Life Sci.* 28: 89–94, 1981.

10. DEVYNCK, M. A., AND P. MEYER. Plasma sodium pump inhibitor in essential hypertension. Relation with sodium intake and hypertensive heredity. In: *Individual Susceptibility to Salt Intake and Arterial Hypertension*, edited by S. Ghione. The Hague, The Netherlands: Koninblijki, 1984, p. 149–158.

12. DIETZ, J. R. Release of atrial natriuretic factor from rat heart-lung preparation by atrial distension. *Am. J. Physiol.* 247 (*Regulatory Integrative Comp. Physiol.* 16): R1093–R1096, 1984.

13. DLOUHA, H., AND M. J. MCBROOM. Atrial natriuretic factor in taurine-treated normal and cardiomyopathic hamsters. *Proc. Soc. Exp. Biol. Med.* 181: 411–415, 1986.

14. EPSTEIN, M. Renal effects of head-out water immersion in man: implications for an understanding of volume homeostasis. *Physiol. Rev.* 58: 529–581, 1978.

15. EPSTEIN, M. Natriuretic hormone and the sodium retention of cirrhosis. *Gastroenterology* 81: 395–397, 1981.

16. ESPINEL, C. Prevention of arterial hypertension in chronic renal failure (abstr.). *Clin. Res.* 23: 35A, 1976.

17. FAVRE, H. Role of the natriuretic factor in the disorders of sodium balance. In: *Advances in Nephrology*, edited by J. Hamburger, J. Crosnier, and M. H. Maxwell. Chicago, IL: Year Book, 1981, vol. 11, p. 3–23.

18. FREEMAN, R. H., K. M. VERBURG, R. C. VARI, D. VILLARREAL, AND J. O. DAVIS. The effect of expansion and depletion of intravascular volume on plasma atrial natriuretic factor levels in the conscious dog (abstr.). *Federation Proc.* 45: 527, 1986.

19. FRIED, T. A., A. T. LAU, M. A. AYON, AND J. H. STEIN. Elevation of ANP levels in ureteral obstruction in the rat (abstr.). *Clin. Res.* 34: 204A, 1986.

20. FRIED, T. A., A. T. LAU, M. A. AYON, AND J. H. STEIN. 28 Amino acid alpha-rANP may not be the peptide released in response to volume expansion in the rat (abstr.). *Clin. Res.* 34: 228A, 1986.

21. GARCIA, R., J. GUTKOWSKA, J. GENEST, M. CANTIN, AND G. THIBAULT. Reduction of blood pressure and increased diuresis and natriuresis during chronic infusion of atrial natriuretic factor (ANF Arg 101-Tyr 126) in conscious one-kidney, one-clip hypertensive rats. *Proc. Soc. Exp. Biol. Med.* 179: 539–545, 1985.

22. GARCIA, R., C. THIBAULT, J. GUTKOWSKA, M. CANTIN, AND J. GENEST. Atrial natriuretic factor and experimental hypertension: a causal role? (abstr.). *Federation Proc.* 44: 1556, 1985.

23. GERBES, A. L., R. M. ARENDT, D. RITTER, D. JÜNGST, J. ZÄHRINGER, AND G. PAUMGARTNER. Plasma atrial natriuretic factor in patients with cirrhosis (Letter to the editor). *N. Engl. J. Med.* 313: 1609–1610, 1985.

24. GRANGER, J. P., J. C. BURNETT, JR., J. C. ROMERO, J. SALAZAR, AND M. JOYCE. Temporal changes in plasma atrial natriuretic peptide during aldosterone escape (abstr.). *Federation Proc.* 45: 527, 1986.

25. GRAVES, S. W., AND G. H. WILLIAMS. An endogenous ouabain-like factor associated with hypertensive pregnant women. *J. Clin. Endocrinol. Metab.* 59: 1070–1074, 1984.

26. GREKIN, R. J., W. D. LING, Y. SHENKER, AND D. F. BOHR. Plasma levels of immunoreactive atrial natriuretic factor (IR-ANF) during the development of DOCA hypertension in pigs (abstr.). In: *Annu. Fall Conf. Sci. Sessions, Counc. High Blood Pressure Res., 39th, Cleveland, OH, Sept. 10–20, 1985*, no. 9.

27. GUTKOWSKA, J., K. HORKY, C. LA CHANCE, K. RACZ, R. GARCIA, G. THIBAULT, O. KUCHEL, J. GENEST, AND M. CANTIN. Atrial natriuretic factor in spontaneously hypertensive rats. *Hypertension Dallas.* 8, Suppl. I: I137–I140, 1986.

28. GUTKOWSKA, J., E. L. SCHIFFRIN, M. CANTIN, AND J. GENEST. Effect of dietary sodium on plasma concentration of immunoreactive atrial natriuretic factor in normal humans (abstr.). *Circulation* 72, Suppl. III: I294, 1985.

29. HADDY, F. J. Local control of vascular resistance as related to hypertension. *Arch. Intern. Med.* 133: 916–931, 1974.

30. HADDY, F. J. Mechanism, prevention and therapy of sodium-dependent hypertension. *Am. J. Med.* 69: 746–758, 1980.

31. HADDY, F. J., AND H. W. OVERBECK. The role of humoral agents in volume expanded hypertension. *Life Sci.* 19: 935–947, 1976.

32. HADDY, F. J., AND M. B. PAMNANI. Evidence for a circulating endogenous Na^+-K^+ pump inhibitor in low-renin hypertension. *Federation Proc.* 44: 2789–2794, 1985.

33. HAMLYN, J. M., P. D. LEVINSON, R. RINGEL, P. A. LEVIN, B. P. HAMILTON, M. P. BLAUSTEIN, AND A. A. KOWARSKI. Relationships among endogenous digitalis-like factors in essential hypertension. *Federation Proc.* 44: 2782–2788, 1985.

34. HILLYARD, S. D., E. LU, AND H. C. GONICK. Further characterization of the natriuretic factor derived from kidney tissue of volume-expanded rats. Effects on short-circuit current and sodium-potassium-adenosine triphosphatase activity. *Circ. Res.* 38: 250–255, 1976.

35. HIRATA, Y., M. GANGULI, L. TOBIAN, AND J. IWAI. Dahl S rats have increased natriuretic factor in the atria but are markedly hyporesponsive to it. *Hypertension Dallas* 6, Suppl. I: I148–I155, 1984.

36. HOLLISTER, A. S., I. TANAKA, J. ONROT, I. BLAGGIONI, AND T. INAGAMI. Modulation of plasma atrial natriuretic factor levels in human subjects by sodium loading and posture change (abstr.). *Circulation* 72, Suppl. III: III102, 1985.

37. HOMCY, C., R. GAIVIN, J. ZISFEIN, AND R. M. GRAHAM. Snack-induced release of atrial natriuretic factor (Letter to the editor). *N. Engl. J. Med.* 313: 1484, 1985.

38. HUOT, S. J., M. B. PAMNANI, D. L. CLOUGH, J. BUGGY, H. J. BRYANT, D. R. HARDER, AND F. J. HADDY. Sodium-potassium pump activity in reduced renal-mass hypertension. *Hypertension Dallas* 5, Suppl. I: I94–I100, 1983.

39. HUOT, S. J., M. B. PAMNANI, D. L. CLOUGH, AND F. J. HADDY. The role of sodium intake, the Na^+-K^+ pump and a ouabain-like humoral agent in the genesis of reduced renal mass hypertension. *Am. J. Nephrol.* 3: 92–99, 1983.

40. KABLITZ, C., R. BARANOWSKI, AND C. WESTENFELDER. Atrial natriuretic peptide levels in a patient prior to and following implantation of an artificial heart (abstr.). *Clin. Res.* 34: 83A, 1986.

41. KIHARA, M., M. KIHARA, AND E. L. BRAVO. Plasma, atrial and brain concentrations of atrial natriuretic polypeptide in unanesthetized mineralocorticoid-hypertensive rats (abstr.). *Federation Proc.* 45: 755, 1986.

42. KOJIMA, I. Circulating digitalis-like substance is increased in DOCA-salt hypertension. *Biochem. Biophys. Res. Commun.* 122: 129–136, 1984.

43. KOLLER, P. T., J. M. NICKLAS, L. A. DI CARLO, Y. SHENKER, AND R. J. GREKIN. Marked elevation of plasma atrial natriuretic factor during paroxysmal supraventricular tachycardia (abstr.). *Circulation* 72, Suppl. III: III102, 1985.

44. KRAMER, H. Natriuretic hormone—its possible role in fluid and electrolyte disturbances in chronic liver disease. *Postgrad. Med. J.* 51: 532–540, 1975.

45. KRAMER, H. J. Antinatriferic and natriuretic activities in human plasma following acute and chronic salt loading. In: *Natriuretic Hormone*, edited by H. J. Kramer and F. Krüick. Berlin: Springer-Verlag, 1978, p. 24–33.

46. KRAMER, H. J., AND H. C. GONICK. Effect of extracellular volume expansion on renal Na-K-ATPase and cell metabolism. *Nephron* 12: 281–296, 1974.

47. LANG, R. E., H. THÖLKEN, D. GANTEN, F. C. LUFT, H. RUSKOAHO, AND T. UNGER. Atrial natriuretic factor—a circulating hormone stimulated by volume loading. *Nature Lond.* 314: 264–266, 1985.

48. LEDSOME, J. R., N. WILSON, C. A. COURNEYA, AND A. F. RANKIN. Release of atrial natriuretic peptide by atrial distension. *Can. J. Physiol. Pharmacol.* 63: 739–742, 1985.

49. LINK, W. T., M. B. PAMNANI, AND F. J. HADDY. Atrial natriuretic factor (ANF) in Dahl strain of hypertensive (HT) and normotensive (NT) rats: effects of dietary salt (abstr.). *Physiologist* 27: 283, 1984.

50. LINK, W. T., M. B. PAMNANI, S. J. HUOT, AND F. J. HADDY. Effect of atrial extract on vascular Na$^+$-K$^+$ pump activity (abstr.). *Physiologist* 24(4): 59, 1981.

51. MATSUO, H., AND K. KANGAWA. Human and rat atrial natriuretic polypeptides and their precursors (abstr.). In: *Int. Symp. Rats Spontaneous Hypertension Related Studies, 5th, Kyoto, Japan, Oct. 20–22, 1985*, p. 104.

52. MCKENZIE, J. C., I. TANAKA, T. INAGAMI, K. S. MISONO, AND R. M. KLEIN. Alterations in atrial and plasma atrial natriuretic factor content during development of hypoxia-induced pulmonary hypertension in the rat. *Proc. Soc. Exp. Biol. Med.* 181: 459–463, 1986.

53. MORII, N., K. NAKAO, M. KIHARA, A. SUGAWARA, M. SAKAMOTO, M. MANO, M. KIHARA, M. SUDA, Y. YAMORI, AND H. IMURA. Decreased left atrial content and increased plasma level of atrial natriuretic polypeptide in SHR and SHR stroke prone (abstr.). In: *Int. Symp. Rats Spontaneous Hypertension Related Studies, 5th, Kyoto, Japan, Oct. 20–22, 1985*, p. 153.

54. NACCARATO, R., P. MESSA, A. D'ANGELO, A. FABRIS, M. MESSA, M. CHIARAMONTE, C. GREGOLIN, AND G. ZANON. Renal handling of sodium and water in early chronic liver disease. Evidence for a reduced natriuretic activity of the cirrhotic urinary extracts in rats. *Gastroenterology* 81: 205–210, 1981.

55. NAKAOKA, H., K. IMATAKA, M. AMANO, J. FUJII, M. ISHIBASHI, AND T. YAMAJI. Plasma levels of atrial natriuretic factor in patients with congestive heart failure (Letter to the editor). *N. Engl. J. Med.* 313: 892–893, 1985.

56. OGIHARA, T., J. KAWASAKI, Y. TABUCHI, K. HASHIZUME, Y. KUMAHARA, K. KANGAWA, AND H. MATSUO. Changes in plasma atrial natriuretic polypeptide (ANP) concentration during head-out water immersion and saline infusion in normal man (abstr.). In: *Annu. Fall Conf. Sci. Sessions, Counc. High Blood Pressure Res., 39th, Cleveland, OH, Sept. 10–20, 1985*, no. 7.

57. OVERBECK, H. W., M. B. PAMNANI, T. AKERA, T. M. BRODY, AND F. J. HADDY. Depressed function of a ouabain-sensitive sodium-potassium pump in blood vessels from renal hypertensive dogs. *Circ. Res.* 38, Suppl. 2: 48–52, 1976.

58. PAGANELLI, W. C., R. R. PINTAL, R. E. COTTER, K. KIFOR, J. R. CANT, AND V. J. DZAU. Influence of acute changes in atrial pressures on plasma atrial natriuretic factor in the conscious dog (abstr.). *Federation Proc.* 45: 754, 1986.

59. PAMNANI, M. B., J. S. CHEN, D. L. CLOUGH, W. T. LINK, AND F. J. HADDY. Rats with reduced renal mass-saline hypertension have increased atrial natriuretic factor. The humoral sodium transport inhibitory factor and atrial natriuretic factor are not the same (abstr.). In: *Sci. Meet. Int. Soc. Hypertension, 10th, Interlaken, Switzerland, June 17–21, 1984*, no. 678.

60. PAMNANI, M. B., D. L. CLOUGH, J. S. CHEN, W. T. LINK, AND F. J. HADDY. Effects of rat atrial extract on sodium transport and blood pressure in the rat. *Proc. Soc. Exp. Biol. Med.* 176: 123–131, 1984.

61. PAMNANI, M., D. CLOUGH, S. HUOT, AND F. HADDY. Sodium-potassium pump activity in experimental hypertension. In: *Vasodilatation*, edited by P. M. Vanhoutte and I. Leusen. New York: Raven, 1981, p. 391–403.

62. PAMNANI, M., S. HUOT, J. BUGGY, D. CLOUGH, AND F. HADDY. Demonstration of a humoral inhibitor of the Na$^+$-K$^+$ pump in some models of experimental hypertension. *Hypertension Dallas* 3, Suppl. II: II96–II101, 1981.

63. PAMNANI, M., S. HUOT, M. JAGUSIAK, W. LINK, AND F. J. HADDY. Effect of atrial extract on hemodynamics in rats (abstr.). *Physiologist* 25: 330, 1982.

64. PAMNANI, M., G. MUELLER, G. HOM, J. SCHOOLEY, AND F. HADDY. Role of atrial natriuretic factor in the development of hypertension in reduced renal mass saline drinking rats (abstr.). *Federation Proc.* 45: 894, 1986.

65. PETTERSSON, A., S.-E. RICKSTEN, A. TOWLE, J. HEDNER, AND T. HEDNER. On the role of atrial natriuretic peptide (ANP) in cardiovascular regulation in SHR (abstr.). In: *Int. Symp. Rats Spontaneous Hypertension Related Studies, 5th, Kyoto, Japan, Oct. 20–22, 1985*, p. 192.

66. PITCOCK, J. A., P. S. BROWN, B. BROOKS, W. L. CLAPP, W. L. BROSIUS, AND E. E. MUIRHEAD. Renomedullary deficiency in partial nephrectomy-salt hypertension. *Hypertension Dallas* 2: 281–290, 1980.

67. POLLOCK, D. M., AND R. O. BANKS. Influence of dietary sodium on the natriuretic activity of atrial tissue. *Miner. Electrolyte Metab.* 10: 337–342, 1984.

68. RAINE, A. E. G., F. B. MÜLLER, R. M. L. BROUWER, E. BÜRGISSER, P. BOLLI, AND F. R.

BÜHLER. Influence of salt balance on plasma levels of atrial natriuretic factor, renin and noradrenaline in man. *J. Hypertens.* 3: 663, 1985.

69. RAPP, J. P., R. M. SNAJDAR, AND H. DENE. Atrial natriuretic factor in inbred Dahl rats (abstr.). In: *Int. Symp. Rats Spontaneous Hypertension Related Studies, 5th, Kyoto, Japan, Oct. 20–22, 1985*, p. 195.

70. SALAZAR, F. J., J. GRANGER, M. JOYCE, AND J. C. ROMERO. Release of atrial natriuretic peptide during plasma osmolality induced increases in vasopressin (abstr.). *Federation Proc.* 45: 528, 1986.

71. SCHIEBINGER, R. J., AND J. M. LINDEN. The influence of stretch and rate of contraction on ANF secretion by rat atria in vitro (abstr.). In: *Ann. Fall Conf. Sci. Sessions, Counc. High Blood Pressure Res., 39th, Cleveland, OH, Sept. 18–20, 1985*, no. 41.

72. SCHIFFRIN, E. L., J. GUTKOWSKA, O. KUCHEL, M. CANTIN, AND J. GENEST. Plasma concentration of atrial natriuretic factor in a patient with paroxysmal atrial tachycardia (Letter to the editor). *N. Engl. J. Med.* 312: 1196–1197, 1985.

73. SCHMIDT, R., J. BOURGOIGNIE, AND N. BRICKER. On the adaptation in sodium excretion in chronic uremia. The effects of proportional reduction of sodium intake. *J. Clin. Invest.* 53: 1736–1741, 1974.

74. SEWELL, R. B., R. D. HUGHES, L. POSTON, AND R. WILLIAMS. Effects of serum from patients with fulminant hepatic failure on leucocyte sodium transport. *Clin. Sci. Lond.* 63: 237–242, 1982.

75. SHENKER, Y., F. K. PORT, M. D. GROSS, R. D. SWARTZ, AND R. J. GREKIN. Plasma levels of immunoreactive atrial natriuretic factor are elevated in patients with end stage renal failure (abstr.). *Clin. Res.* 33: 895A, 1985.

75a. SHENKER, Y., R. S. SIDER, E. A. OSTAFIN, AND R. J. GREKIN. Plasma levels of immunoreactive atrial natriuretic factor in healthy subjects and in patients with edema. *J. Clin. Invest.* 76: 1684–1687, 1985.

76. SONGU-MIZE, E., S. L. BEALER, AND R. W. CALDWELL. Effect of AV3V lesions on development of DOCA-salt hypertension and vascular Na^+-pump activity. *Hypertension Dallas* 4: 575–580, 1982.

77. SONNENBERG, H., S. MILOJEVIC, C. K. CHONG, AND A. T. VERESS. Atrial natriuretic factor: reduced cardiac content in spontaneously hypertensive rats. *Hypertension Dallas* 5: 672–675, 1983.

78. STRUTHERS, A. D., J. V. ANDERSON, N. PAYNE, J. D. H. SLATER, AND S. R. BLOOM. Atrial natriuretic peptide inhibits the aldosterone response to angiotensin II in man. *J. Hypertens.* 3: 662–663, 1985.

79. SUZUKI, H., H. SANO, K. KARIYA, K. SAITO, Y. FURUTA, AND J. YAMANISHI. Plasma Na-K-ATPase inhibitor and erythrocyte sodium transport in uremia (abstr.). *Circulation* 72, Suppl. III: III214, 1985.

80. TANAKA, I., AND T. INAGAMI. Increased plasma concentration of plasma immunoreactive atrial natriuretic factor in Dahl salt sensitive rats with sodium chloride-induced hypertension. *J. Hypertens.* 4: 109–112, 1986.

80a. TANAKA, I., K. S. MISONO, AND T. INAGAMI. Atrial natriuretic factor in rat hypothalamus, atria and plasma: determination by specific radioimmunoassay. *Biochem. Biophys. Res. Commun.* 124: 663–668, 1984.

81. THIBAULT, G., R. GARCIA, M. CANTIN, AND J. GENEST. Atrial natriuretic factor. Characterization and partial purification. *Hypertension Dallas* 5, Suppl. I: I75–I80, 1983.

82. TIKKANEN, I., F. FYHRQUIST, K. METSÄRINNE, AND R. LEIDENIUS. Plasma atrial natriuretic peptide in cardiac disease and during infusion in healthy volunteers. *Lancet* 2: 66–69, 1985.

82a. WARDENER, H. E. DE, AND E. M. CLARKSON. Concept of natriuretic hormone. *Physiol. Rev.* 65: 659–759, 1985.

83. VALDES, R., JR. Endogenous digoxin-immunoreactive factor in human subjects. *Federation Proc.* 44: 2800–2805, 1985.

84. VARI, R. C., K. M. VERBURG, D. VILLARREAL, J. O. DAVIS, AND R. H. FREEMAN. Changes in plasma atrial natriuretic factor in rats after volume expansion or after synthetic ANF infusion (abstr.). *Federation Proc.* 45: 527, 1986.

85. VILLARREAL, D., K. M. VERBURG, R. C. VARI, J. O. DAVIS, AND R. H. FREEMAN. Release of atrial natriuretic factor in dogs with experimental high output heart failure (abstr.). *Federation Proc.* 45: 527, 1986.

86. YAMAJI, T., M. ISHIBASHI, H. NAKAOKA, K. IMATAKA, M. AMANO, AND J. FUJII. Possible role

for atrial natriuretic peptide in polyuria associated with paroxysmal atrial arrhythmias. *Lancet* 1: 1211, 1985.

87. YAMAJI, T., M. ISHIBASHI, AND F. TAKAKU. Atrial natriuretic factor in human blood. *J. Clin. Invest.* 76: 1705–1709, 1985.

88. YANDLE, T. G., I. CROZIER, E. A. ESPINER, H. IKRAM, AND M. G. NICHOLLS. Production, plasma levels, and clearance of atrial natriuretic peptides in man (abstr.). In: *Annu. Fall Conf. Sci. Sessions, Counc. High Blood Pressure Res., 39th, Sept. 10–20, 1985,* no. 8.

89. YASUHARA, S., I. MIYAMORI, T. MORISE, S. OKAMOTO, AND R. TAKEDA. Urinary digitalis-like substance in spontaneously hypertensive rat (abstr.). In: *Int. Symp. Rats Spontaneous Hypertension Related Studies, 5th, Kyoto, Japan, Oct. 20–22, 1985,* p. 158.

90. YLITALO, P., AND F. GROSS. Hemodynamic changes during the development of sodium-induced hypertension in subtotally nephrectomized rats. *Acta Physiol. Scand.* 106: 447–455, 1979.

91. YLITALO, P., R. HEPP, J. MÖHRING, P. OSTER, AND F. GROSS. Effects of varying sodium intake on blood pressure and renin-angiotensin system in subtotally nephrectomized rats. *J. Lab. Clin. Med.* 88: 807–816, 1976.

INDEX